Breast Ultrasound

Guest Editor

GARY J. WHITMAN, MD

ULTRASOUND CLINICS

www.ultrasound.theclinics.com

Consulting Editor
VIKRAM S. DOGRA, MD

July 2011 • Volume 6 • Number 3

SAUNDERS an imprint of ELSEVIER, Inc.

W.B. SAUNDERS COMPANY
A Division of Elsevier Inc.

1600 John F. Kennedy Boulevard • Suite 1800 • Philadelphia, Pennsylvania 19103-2899

http://www.theclinics.com

ULTRASOUND CLINICS Volume 6, Number 3
July 2011 ISSN 1556-858X, ISBN-13: 978-1-4557-0515-3

Editor: Barton Dudlick

Ultrasound Clinics (ISSN 1556-858X) is published quarterly by W.B. Saunders, 360 Park Avenue South, New York, NY 10010-1710. Months of publication are January, April, July, and October. Business and editorial offices: 1600 John F. Kennedy Boulevard, Suite 1800, Philadelphia, Pennsylvania 19103-2899. Accounting and circulation offices: 6277 Sea Harbor Drive, Orlando, FL 32887-4800. Periodicals postage paid at New York, NY, and additional mailing offices. Subscription prices are $225 per year for (US individuals), $279 per year for (US institutions), $107 per year for (US students and residents), $253 per year for (Canadian individuals), $312 per year for (Canadian institutions), $269 per year for (international individuals), $312 per year for (international institutions), and $129 per year for (Canadian and foreign students/residents). To receive student/resident rate, orders must be accompanied by name of affiliated institution, date of term, and the signature of program/residency coordinator on institution letterhead. Orders will be billed at individual rate until proof of status is received. Foreign air speed delivery is included in all Clinics subscription prices. All prices are subject to change without notice. **POSTMASTER:** Send address changes to *Ultrasound Clinics,* Elsevier Health Sciences Division, Subscription Customer Service, 3251 Riverport Lane, Maryland Heights, MO 63043. **Customer Service (orders, claims, online, change of address): Telephone: 1-800-654-2452 (U.S. and Canada); 314-447-8871 (outside U.S. and Canada). Fax: 314-447-8029. E-mail: journalscustomerservice-usa@elsevier.com (for print support); journalsonlinesupport-usa@elsevier.com (for online support).**

Reprints: For copies of 100 or more, of articles in this publication, please contact the Commercial Reprints Department, Elsevier Inc., 360 Park Avenue South, New York, NY 10010-1710. Tel.: (+1) 212-633-3812; Fax: (+1) 212-462-1935; E-mail: reprints@elsevier.com.

Printed and bound by CPI Group (UK) Ltd, Croydon, CR0 4YY

Transferred to Digital Print 2011

Contributors

CONSULTING EDITOR

VIKRAM S. DOGRA, MD
Professor of Radiology, Urology, and
Biomedical Engineering, Director of Ultrasound
and Associate Chair for Education and
Research, Department of Imaging Sciences,
University of Rochester School of Medicine
and Dentistry, Rochester, New York

GUEST EDITOR

GARY J. WHITMAN, MD
Professor of Radiology and Radiation
Oncology, Departments of Diagnostic
Radiology and Radiation Oncology,
The University of Texas MD Anderson
Cancer Center, Houston, Texas

AUTHORS

MARGARET ADEJOLU, MRCP, FRCR
Breast Imaging Fellow, Department
of Radiology, King's College Hospital,
Denmark Hill, London, United Kingdom;
Department of Diagnostic Radiology,
The University of Texas MD Anderson
Cancer Center, Houston, Texas

CHRISTOPHER COMSTOCK, MD
Breast Imaging Service, Department
of Radiology, Memorial Sloan-Kettering
Cancer Center, New York, New York

PHAN T. HUYNH, MD
Medical Director, Department of Radiology,
St Luke's Women Center, St Luke's Episcopal
Hospital, Houston, Texas

SAVITRI KRISHNAMURTHY, MD
Professor of Pathology, Department of
Pathology, The University of Texas MD
Anderson Cancer Center, Houston, Texas

TRACY J. LU
Department of Diagnostic Radiology,
The University of Texas MD Anderson
Cancer Center, Houston, Texas;
Undergraduate Student, Harvard College,
Cambridge, Massachusetts

DENNIS N. MCDONALD, MD
Director, Women's Imaging, Breast Care
Center, Sutter Pacific Medical Foundation,
Santa Rosa, California

MICHAEL P. MCNAMARA Jr, MD
Associate Professor of Radiology, Chief,
Breast Imaging and Intervention, Case School
of Medicine, MetroHealth Medical Center,
Cleveland, Ohio; Adjunct Faculty, Uniformed
Services, University of the Health Sciences,
Bethesda, Maryland

MICHAEL S. MIDDLETON, MD, PhD
Assistant Professor of Radiology,
Department of Radiology, University
of California, San Diego, California

EMILY L. SEDGWICK, MD
Assistant Professor, Director of Breast
Imaging, Department of Radiology,
Baylor College of Medicine, Houston,
Texas

R. JASON STAFFORD, PhD
Department of Imaging Physics, Division
of Diagnostic Imaging, The University
of Texas MD Anderson Cancer Center,
Houston, Texas

DECLAN SHEPPARD, FRCR
Consultant Radiologist, Department of
Radiology, Portiuncula Hospital, Ballinasloe,
Galway, Ireland

GARY J. WHITMAN, MD
Professor of Radiology and Radiation
Oncology, Departments of Diagnostic
Radiology and Radiation Oncology, The
University of Texas MD Anderson Cancer
Center, Houston, Texas

Contents

Preface: Breast Ultrasound   ix

Gary J. Whitman

Ultrasound Physics and Technology in Breast Imaging   299

R. Jason Stafford, PhD and Gary J. Whitman, MD

> Ultrasound is used in breast imaging for differentiation of cysts from solid masses and to provide real-time guidance for interventional procedures. Breast ultrasound plays an integral role in evaluating palpable findings, asymmetric breast tissue, and developing densities. Advances contribute to the role of ultrasound in guiding and facilitating minimally invasive procedures. This article briefly reviews some of the hallmarks of modern ultrasound systems relevant to breast ultrasound, discusses recent advances, and outlines how these advances may affect clinical breast ultrasound diagnostic and interventional procedures.

Ultrasound of Invasive Lobular Carcinoma   313

Margaret Adejolu, Savitri Krishnamurthy, and Gary J. Whitman

> Invasive lobular carcinoma (ILC) is the second most common type of breast malignancy, constituting 4% to 15% of all breast cancers. It is difficult to detect clinically and mammographically. This article reviews the histopathological and the imaging appearances of ILC, with particular emphasis on the appearance of ILC on sonography.

Ultrasound-Guided Breast Biopsy   327

Emily L. Sedgwick

> Since it was originally described in 1993, ultrasound-guided core needle biopsy has been shown to be a reliable, even preferred, alternative to open surgical biopsy. This technique should be the modality of choice for any breast or axillary sonographic abnormality requiring tissue sampling. The high sensitivity and reproducibility of this technique make this technique a low-cost procedure that minimizes patient morbidity. As ultrasound-guided core needle biopsy gains wider acceptance, its therapeutic uses, such as removal of masses, are becoming more prevalent.

Ultrasonography and Ultrasound-Guided Biopsy of Breast Calcifications   335

Phan T. Huynh

> Breast calcifications are frequently identified on mammography in the screening and diagnostic settings. If the indeterminate calcifications are classified as suspicious (Breast Imaging Reporting and Data System [BI-RADS] category 4) or highly suggestive (BI-RADS category 5) of malignancy, histopathological confirmation can be usually accomplished with stereotactic biopsy. This article discusses the increase use of ultrasonography in the evaluation and management of BI-RADS 4 and 5 breast calcifications.

Ultrasound of Breast Implants and Soft Tissue Silicone   345

Michael P. McNamara Jr and Michael S. Middleton

> Ultrasound can detect most implant rupture and is more sensitive than magnetic resonance (MR) imaging in the detection of soft tissue silicone. Rupture detection should be focused mainly on identification of the variable degree of shell collapse that occurs when silicone gel escapes the implant as a whole. Ultrasound evaluation has limitations, so correlation with MRI may be necessary. This article provides the sonographer and sonologist with an overview of normal and abnormal implant findings, reviews the spectrum of appearance of soft tissue silicone, and discusses some pitfalls that can be encountered.

Lymph Node Sonography   369

Gary J. Whitman, Tracy J. Lu, Margaret Adejolu, Savitri Krishnamurthy, and Declan Sheppard

> The sonographic appearances of benign (normal and reactive) and malignant (metastatic and lymphomatous) lymph nodes can be explained by an understanding of normal nodal anatomy and nodal pathophysiology. This article reviews the sonographic features of benign and malignant regional (axillary, infraclavicular, internal mammary, and supraclavicular) lymph nodes. As axillary lymph nodes are those most frequently involved in patients with breast cancer, this review focuses mainly on axillary lymph nodes.

3-Dimensional Breast Ultrasonography: What Have We Been Missing?   381

Dennis N. McDonald

> It is believed that 3-dimensional breast ultrasonography is poised to offer a new paradigm in breast ultrasound imaging by changing the way imaging is carried out, specifically the way breast ultrasound examinations are acquired, reviewed, and interpreted. In this article, we discuss briefly the physics of volume imaging. We also discuss the principles of volume acquisitions, the advantages and limitations of all volume acquisition techniques, and the suggestions for applications in the busy breast imaging practice.

Ultrasound Elastography of Breast Lesions   407

Christopher Comstock

> Static or compressive elastography (ultrasound [US] strain imaging) and acoustic radiation force impulse, of which shear wave elastography is a subtype, are the 2 main methods of breast US elastography and they differ by the type of stress or vibration applied. This article discusses using elastographic information for lesion analysis as an adjunct to the standard gray-scale morphologic and color Doppler information.

Index   417

Ultrasound Clinics

FORTHCOMING ISSUES

October 2011

Vascular Ultrasound
Deborah Rubens, MD, and
Edward G. Grant, MD, *Guest Editors*

January 2012

Obstetric and Gynecologic Ultrasound
Phyllis Glanc MD, FRCPC (C), *Guest Editor*

RECENT ISSUES

April 2011

Emergency Ultrasound
Jill Langer, MD, *Guest Editor*

January 2011

Advanced Obstetric Ultrasound
Theodore Dubinsky, MD, and
Manjiri Dighe, MD, *Guest Editors*

RELATED INTEREST

September 2010
Radiologic Clinics
Breast Imaging
Robyn L. Birdwell, MD, FACR, *Guest Editor*

THE CLINICS ARE NOW AVAILABLE ONLINE!

Access your subscription at:
www.theclinics.com

GOAL STATEMENT

The goal of the *Ultrasound Clinics* is to keep practicing radiologists and radiology residents up to date with current clinical practice in ultrasound by providing timely articles reviewing the state of the art in patient care.

ACCREDITATION

The *Ultrasound Clinics* is planned and implemented in accordance with the Essential Areas and Policies of the Accreditation Council for Continuing Medical Education (ACCME) through the joint sponsorship of the University of Virginia School of Medicine and Elsevier. The University of Virginia School of Medicine is accredited by the ACCME to provide continuing medical education for physicians.

The University of Virginia School of Medicine designates this enduring material activity for a maximum of 15 *AMA PRA Category 1 Credit*(s)™ for each issue, 60 credits per year. Physicians should claim only the credit commensurate with the extent of their participation in the activity.

The American Medical Association has determined that physicians not licensed in the US who participate in this CME activity are eligible for a maximum of 15 *AMA PRA Category 1 Credit*(s)™ for each issue, 60 credits per year.

Credit can be earned by reading the text material, taking the CME examination online at http://www.theclinics.com/home/cme, and completing the evaluation. After taking the test, you will be required to review any and all incorrect answers. Following completion of the test and evaluation, your credit will be awarded and you may print your certificate.

FACULTY DISCLOSURE/CONFLICT OF INTEREST

The University of Virginia School of Medicine, as an ACCME accredited provider, endorses and strives to comply with the Accreditation Council for Continuing Medical Education (ACCME) Standards of Commercial Support, Commonwealth of Virginia statutes, University of Virginia policies and procedures, and associated federal and private regulations and guidelines on the need for disclosure and monitoring of proprietary and financial interests that may affect the scientific integrity and balance of content delivered in continuing medical education activities under our auspices.

The University of Virginia School of Medicine requires that all CME activities accredited through this institution be developed independently and be scientifically rigorous, balanced and objective in the presentation/discussion of its content, theories and practices.

All authors/editors participating in an accredited CME activity are expected to disclose to the readers relevant financial relationships with commercial entities occurring within the past 12 months (such as grants or research support, employee, consultant, stock holder, member of speakers bureau, etc.). The University of Virginia School of Medicine will employ appropriate mechanisms to resolve potential conflicts of interest to maintain the standards of fair and balanced education to the reader. Questions about specific strategies can be directed to the Office of Continuing Medical Education, University of Virginia School of Medicine, Charlottesville, Virginia.

The faculty and staff of the University of Virginia Office of Continuing Medical Education have no financial affiliations to disclose.

The authors/editors listed below have identified no professional or financial affiliations for themselves or their spouse/partner:
Margaret Adejolu, MRCP, FRCR; Christopher Comstock, MD; Barton Dudlick (Acquisitions Editor); Phan T. Huynh, MD; Savitri Krishnamurthy, MD; Tracy J. Lu; Michael P. McNamara Jr, MD; Emily L. Sedgwick, MD; Declan Sheppard, FRCR; R. Jason Stafford, PhD; and Gary J. Whitman (Guest Editor).

The authors/editors listed below have identified the following professional or financial affiliations for themselves or their spouse/partner:
Matthew J. Bassignani, MD (Test Author) is on the Advisory Board/Committee for Nuance and Fuji Medical Systems.
Vikram S. Dogra, MD (Consulting Editor) is the editor for the Journal of Clinical Imaging Science.
Dennis N. McDonald, MD is an industry funded research/investigator and is on the Speaker's Bureau for GE Healthcare.
Michael S. Middleton, MD, PhD is a consultant for Merge/Confirma and Siemens; is an industry funded research/investigator for General Electric, Siemens, and Bayer; owns stock with General Electric; and is on the Speakers' Bureau for Merge/Confirma.

Disclosure of Discussion of Non-FDA Approved Uses for Pharmaceutical Products and/or Medical Devices
The University of Virginia School of Medicine, as an ACCME provider, requires that all faculty presenters identify and disclose any off-label uses for pharmaceutical and medical device products. The University of Virginia School of Medicine recommends that each physician fully review all the available data on new products or procedures prior to clinical use.

TO ENROLL

To enroll in the Ultrasound Clinics Continuing Medical Education program, call customer service at 1-800-654-2452 or visit us online at www.theclinics.com/home/cme. The CME program is available to subscribers for an additional fee of $196.00.

Preface
Breast Ultrasound

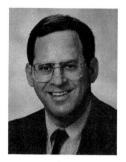

Gary J. Whitman, MD
Guest Editor

As I write this, I am in an airplane, flying home to Houston from a family event in Virginia. To my left, my children, Sam and Kayla, are watching *The Lion King* on a video player, and Susan, my wife, is reading *Cutting for Stone* by Abraham Verghese. To my right, a soldier-turned-civilian is just returning from a State Department assignment in Afghanistan. No doubt he has made a difference.

Leaning back in my seat, I think about breast ultrasound in the middle of 2011. In the last decade, the advances have been remarkable: smaller, faster, more powerful ultrasound units with better resolution and markedly improved image quality. No question. There is a big difference.

In this issue of *Ultrasound Clinics*, we explore selected topics in breast sonography. Jason Stafford and I provide an overview of advances in breast ultrasound physics and technology. Margaret Adejolu, Savitri Krishnamurthy, and I then review the sonographic features of invasive lobular carcinoma. Emily Sedgwick provides a review of ultrasound-guided breast biopsies. Phan Huynh discusses ultrasound and ultrasound-guided biopsy of breast calcifications. Michael McNamara and Michael Middleton review breast implants and soft-tissue silicone. Collaborating with Tracy Lu, Margaret Adejolu, Savitri Krishnamurthy, and Declan Sheppard, I provide an update on lymph node sonography. We conclude this issue with two articles on exciting new applications, three-dimensional breast ultrasound, by Dennis McDonald, and elastography, by Chris Comstock.

I would like to thank all of the authors for a wonderful job, especially when so much of this work gets done at night and on weekends. Kudos to all the authors and coauthors! You have made a difference, and you will continue to make a big difference.

Barbara Almarez Mahinda was a tremendous help (as usual) in manuscript preparation, image preparation, and editing. Joyce Bradley did a great job, helping to prepare several articles. Barbara and Joyce, many thanks!

I want to thank Vikram Dogra for his support. Thanks to Barton Dudlick for all of his organizational help and his patience.

When I think of making a difference, I am drawn to my parents. My mom, Nancy Whitman, is a wonderful mother and role model. She is a steady source of encouragement in my life. My dad, Marvin Whitman, passed away in the fall of 2010, as this issue was being developed. My father was a great man, a skilled obstetrician-gynecologist and a true physician educator. He practiced obstetrics and gynecology, mainly before sonography became an everyday tool. His interest in ultrasound was high as he watched sonography blossom. I thank

Ultrasound Clin 6 (2011) ix–x
doi:10.1016/j.cult.2011.06.001

my parents for helping me and for providing the opportunities that made a big difference for me.

Susan, Sam, and Kayla, I thank you for allowing me to work on this project. I often wandered into my home office to work on *Ultrasound Clinics*. Sometimes, I would leave home a little earlier in the morning or return from work a little later in the evening, trying to carve out time to work on this issue. Susan, Sam, and Kayla, thank you again and again! In my eyes, you are the difference.

Gary J. Whitman, MD
Departments of Diagnostic Radiology and
Radiation Oncology
The University of Texas MD Anderson Cancer Center
Unit 1350
PO Box 301439
Houston, TX 77230-1439, USA

E-mail address:
gwhitman@mdanderson.org

Ultrasound Physics and Technology in Breast Imaging

R. Jason Stafford, PhD[a],*, Gary J. Whitman, MD[b]

KEYWORDS

- Ultrasound • Breast imaging • Cysts • Imaging technology

Ultrasound is an inexpensive, portable, nonionizing, real-time imaging modality. Ultrasound is commonly used in breast imaging for differentiation of cysts from solid masses and to provide real-time guidance for interventional procedures.[1,2] It has been nearly 10 years since digital broadband ultrasound systems became widely available. During this time, considerable advances in image acquisition and reconstruction have taken advantage of this paradigm shift in ultrasound system design to enhance resolution, contrast, and penetration. Ultrasound imaging technology continues to remain in a state of rapid flux as innovations and refinements in technology continue to be introduced.

New applications and enhancements in image quality have significantly influenced the role of ultrasound in clinical imaging. These findings are particularly true with respect to diagnosis and interventions in the breast, where these advancements, in conjunction with a standardized reporting system (Breast Imaging Reporting and Data System [BI-RADS]),[3,4] have enabled breast ultrasound to progress beyond its previous role into the realm of ascertaining the probability of malignancy for solid masses. In addition, breast ultrasound plays an integral role in the evaluation of palpable findings, asymmetric breast tissue, and developing densities. Many recent advances are also contributing to the expanding role of ultrasound in guiding and facilitating more minimally invasive procedures.

Although a detailed review of clinical breast sonography is beyond the scope of this technology-oriented overview, interest continues to mount in applying breast ultrasound as a secondary screening tool.[5] A single-center retrospective screening trial indicated that ultrasound may be useful for evaluating women who present with dense parenchyma on mammography, palpable findings on physical examination, and suspicious mammographic findings.[6] A multicenter blinded study investigating the use of ultrasound as a secondary screening modality along with mammography (ACRIN 6666) found that ultrasound identified additional cancers not seen on mammography, at the expense of generating false-positive results, thus generally increasing the number of interventions performed.[7] Therefore, as ultrasound continues to advance, to minimize the amount of unnecessary interventions, there is a need to increase the specificity of breast ultrasound as well as the sensitivity.

Given the rapid technologic change, it can often be difficult to discern between claims made for marketing purposes versus true advancements when it comes to ultrasound technology.[8] The goal of this article is to provide a brief review of some of the hallmarks of modern ultrasound systems relevant to breast ultrasound, discuss recent advances, and outline how these advances may affect clinical breast ultrasound diagnostic and interventional procedures.

[a] Department of Imaging Physics, Division of Diagnostic Imaging, The University of Texas MD Anderson Cancer Center, 1515 Holcombe Boulevard, Unit 056, Houston, TX 77030, USA
[b] Departments of Diagnostic Radiology and Radiation Oncology, The University of Texas MD Anderson Cancer Center, Unit 1350, PO Box 301439, Houston, TX 77230-1439, USA
* Corresponding author.
E-mail address: jstafford@mdanderson.org

Ultrasound Clin 6 (2011) 299–312
doi:10.1016/j.cult.2011.02.001
1556-858X/11/$ – see front matter © 2011 Elsevier Inc. All rights reserved.

BREAST ULTRASOUND SYSTEM ARCHITECTURE AND DESIGN

Owing to miniaturization of key electronic components, current ultrasound systems are smaller, lighter, and more ergonomically optimized than previous systems. The knobs and dials that sonographers have grown accustomed to tend to remain on the systems in similar locations to maintain a sense of familiarity, but in many cases, the functionality of the individual buttons and knobs has been expanded to facilitate easy access to some of the common real-time options. Touch screens are often incorporated into the systems to gain access to additional options, such as filters or 3-D functionality.

Modern systems optimized for breast imaging applications tend to be fully digital, providing an independent channel to each element with its own analog-to-digital converter (ADC) and preamplifier. Ultra–low noise preamplifiers have aided in the improvement of dynamic range and penetration with signal digitization occurring immediately afterwards. Digital integrated circuit technology aids in miniaturization of the electronics, keeping transducers light and facilitating designs that can accommodate ergonomic concerns.

Due to the advances in computational processing power in conjunction with the design of these fully digital systems,[9] many features that have remained static for many years, such as transmit gain control (TGC), are evolving. On analog systems, TGC is implemented by manual adjustments of 6 to 9 sliding dashpots on the ultrasound console, which adjust the gain in different zones to compensate for beam attenuation as a function of depth, providing a more uniform image. Applying TGC before ADC reduced the dynamic range and facilitated the use of lower performance ADC devices. Increasingly, state-of-the-art systems are implementing TGC after digitization, facilitating automated gain adjustment features that free up sonographers' time. Some implementations also provide adjustment of the horizontal gain in sectors to further enhance image uniformity. Some more fully digital systems apply TGC after the signal has been digitized. These factors can facilitate retrospective manual or automatic optimization of the gain, even when the image is frozen. On these systems, many factors may be adjusted manually or automatically after the image is frozen, including compression (the amount of logarithmic dynamic range adjustment applied to the signal). This trend in using image analysis and feedback from the ultrasound system to automatically optimize acquisitions is quickly maturing and expanding to optimize parameters associated with other acquisitions, such as Doppler sonography.

More importantly, modern systems enable the use of digital beamforming, which is highly programmable. Digital beamforming, in conjunction with broadband transducer technology and fast, dedicated digital signal processing, has been the key enabling technology for many advanced transmit and acquisition techniques that were not feasible a few years ago.

Electronic control of beamforming facilitates independent modulation of each element used in the excitation and receive aperture and the use of much larger and precise timing delays for beam steering and focusing than analog electronics could provide. These improvements have facilitated the use of larger apertures to obtain better lateral resolution as well as adaptively weighted excitation of the elements of the aperture (apodization) to minimize side lobes and grating lobes generated by beam steering. Used in conjunction with the broad bandwidth of modern transducers, dynamic receive apertures facilitate increased penetration and more uniform resolution by using the high frequencies in the near field combined with smaller receive apertures and larger apertures for the more penetrating lower frequencies. Additionally, parallel acquisition techniques may be used to increase frame rates or resolution by using a large aperture for excitation and several smaller, overlapped apertures for receiving multiple delayed A lines. Such technology may be useful in enhancing 3-D or 4-D imaging techniques. Broadband digital beamforming also facilitates modern acquisition techniques, such as spatial and frequency compounding and tissue harmonic imaging.

Although the peak acoustic output is currently limited by Food and Drug Administration regulations, a successful method for increasing the penetration of the ultrasound beam has been coded excitation technology.[10,11] Although short, high-pressure, ultrasound excitation pulses are normally essential for high-resolution imaging, coded excitation technology is able to use longer pulse trains, with specific digital amplitude or frequency modulation, to deliver more energy without raising the peak acoustic pressure. Although a potential for artifacts exists, resolution is recovered via digital demodulation and filtering of the beam, enabling higher-frequency imaging without loss of penetration as well as increased quality of Doppler and harmonic imaging.[12]

Ultrasound Probes

In addition to the increases in sensitivity brought about by digital beamformer design, better front-end electronics and coded excitation and advances in transducer array material design that have an impact on sensitivity, such as increased electromechanical coupling and lowered acoustic impedance, have helped enable a move to higher frequencies.[13,14] For optimal axial and lateral resolution, modern probes for breast ultrasound have generally increased in frequency, with frequencies in excess of 10 MHz considered standard, and new probes have bandwidths in excess of 18 MHz. Axial resolution is further enhanced by the wide bandwidth of these transducers.[15] Despite the higher frequencies, these transducers can have bandwidths in excess of 150% (heavily damped, short ultrasound pulses). These broadband transducers also facilitate many of the modern image contrast solutions in ultrasound, such as tissue harmonic imaging and frequency compounding.

Lateral resolution is further enhanced by an increased number of transducer probe elements. There are at least 500 elements on many modern high-resolution linear transducers used in breast ultrasound. The increased number of independent elements is also used to mitigate side lobes as well as grating lobes associated with beam steering. The amplitude pattern of the transmit aperture can be electronically modulated to reduce these artifacts, leading to potentially less clutter.

Of particular relevance to breast ultrasound has been the increase in the number of elements in the elevational direction. These multirow or 1.5-D high-frequency transducers have enough elements for dynamic electronic focusing in the elevational direction to improve both slice thickness and sensitivity at depth, allowing visualization of deeper structures in the breast.[16] An alternative approach that does not require additional elements is the Hanafy lens.[17] This variation on the traditional mechanical lens actually varies the thickness of the ceramic of each transducer element as well as electronically modulating the approach to transmit/receive, to achieve a similar affect.

The impact of wielding transducers with increased numbers of elements and independent channels has been mitigated by the move to digital electronics and integrated circuits, which keeps the weight of the transducer low, and by benefits from advances in ergonomic design.

Extended Field-of-View Imaging

With increases in frame rate, real-time processing, and storage, the ability to extend the field of view beyond the footprint of the transducer has arisen by storing images in real time and applying pattern recognition while an operator slides the transducer along the direction desired, extending the field of view with a free-hand technique (**Fig. 1**). Over the

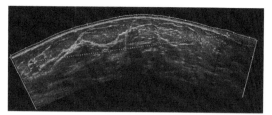

Fig. 1. EFV imaging. By moving the transducer along the direction of the field of view, EFV imaging can be used to visualize findings in relation to breast landmarks. Additionally, accurate measurements can be made. The cursors indicate the distance from the cyst to the nipple.

past decade, use of extended field-of-view (EFV) imaging has become ubiquitous in breast ultrasound[18] because it can be used for accurately[19] assessing the distance between structures and findings in the breast beyond the 2-D field of view of the ultrasound probe, including analysis of the nodal basins, large scars and seromas, and multifocal and multicentric disease. In addition, EFV imaging is often used for documentation of the distance between the lesion and the nipple. Information from EFV sonograms is useful for surgical planning as well as for diagnostic evaluation of the breast. Commercial implementation of this technique goes by many names (**Table 1**). Currently, many systems allow advanced contrast

Table 1
Some standard and emerging technologies available on commercial scanners

Ultrasound Technology	Example Commercial Names
Phase aberration correction	Tissue Aberration Correction, Fatty Tissue Imaging
Spatial compounding	SonoCT, SieClear, CrossBeam, ApliPure, HI Compound
Real-time speckle processing	XRES, Dynamic Tissue Contrast Enhancement, Speckle Reduction Imaging
EFV imaging	Panoramic Imaging, Siescape, LOGIQView, FreeStyle Extended Imaging, ApliClear
Elastography	
Static	Elastography, eSieTouch, SonoElastography
Acoustic force radiation impulse	Shear Wave Elasticity Imaging, Virtual Touch

modes, such as tissue harmonic imaging and spatial compounding, as well as duplex modes, such as power doppler (PD), when acquiring an EFV image (see **Fig. 1**).

3-D/4-D Imaging

If an ultrasound probe is dragged in the elevational direction with a free-hand technique, most modern systems have enough memory to buffer these images so that a cine of the multiple slices captured can be saved to a disk for review of the volume. By applying approaches similar to those used in EFV to pattern recognition, often with the assistance of motion sensors in the probes, a 3-D volume can be acquired using free-hand technique. Unfortunately, free-hand techniques are limited in reproducibility and in the ability to perform dynamic volume acquisitions (4-D imaging). To address this limitation, vendors have moved beyond 1.5-D probes to fully 2-D probes, with thousands of elements, capable of electronic beam steering in the elevational direction for rapid 3-D and 4-D imaging. This approach is still not suitable, however, for screening the entire breast.

Interest in applying this technology to breast ultrasound, potentially as a screening tool, has prompted several vendors to develop dedicated systems with large numbers of arrays on articulating arms for easy, reproducible scanning across the entire breast. This technology allows high-resolution coronal images of the breast to be reconstructed and evaluated in addition to axial and sagittal images. Similar to how MRI collects multiple tissue contrast images, in the future, this technology is likely to be coupled with one or more of the multiple contrast mechanisms being investigated in breast ultrasound, such as tissue harmonic imaging, spatial compounding, PD imaging, and, potentially, dynamic contrast-enhanced imaging. Currently, researchers are evaluating the role, artifacts, and limitations of 3-D imaging in diagnostic breast ultrasound and analyzing 3-D imaging's role in surgical planning and guidance for interventional procedures.[20]

SPEED OF SOUND CORRECTION

The average speed of sound in soft tissue is often assumed to be close to 1540 m/s for range calculations for distance and focusing by the beamformer. Unfortunately, the lower speed of sound in fatty tissue (1450 m/s) tends to reduce this average. These findings result in geometric inaccuracies because of differences in the speed of sound in adipose tissue and soft tissue.[21] More relevant to imaging in the breast, these timing errors also have a detrimental impact on image

quality.[22,23] All lateral and elevational beam focusing and steering are accomplished via time shifts, which are calibrated using the estimated speed of sound. Phase aberrations are the errors in focusing caused by the incorrect estimation of the speed of sound, and these errors lead to reduced resolution, reduced beam penetration, and a distortion of the speckle pattern.[24] Such image quality losses are exacerbated in imaging of breasts with a substantial amount of fatty tissue and are much less noticeable in breasts consisting of dense fibroglandular tissue.

Although investigations of techniques for phase aberration correction date back to the 1970s, the commercial implementation of this technology is still new. Many modern, state-of-the-art ultrasound scanners are beginning to incorporate first-generation phase aberration correction into their systems, usually implemented as an imaging option that can be turned on or off. These corrections are of particular value in breast ultrasound in that the ability to better visualize groups of calcifications and subtle distortions is likely to be enhanced in many instances,[25] similar to what investigations in phantoms predict (**Fig. 2**).[26] Phase aberration correction was not implemented during the most recent multicenter trials involving the use of ultrasound as a secondary screening modality nor has it been evaluated when used in conjunction with speckle reduction or tissue harmonic imaging techniques (described later). In an era where the BI-RADS lexicon[3,4] for ultrasound is available, the potentially subtle impact of this technology on the description of findings in the breast (**Fig. 3**) should likely be evaluated systematically and not left to anecdotal observations or conjectures by vendors as to its appropriate use.

SPECKLE REDUCTION

Speckle is the name given to the granular-appearing background noise that is the result of coherent interference with ultrasound waves.[27] Additional sources of noise and artifacts that confound ultrasound interpretation include clutter (spurious signals generated from objects not in the primary beam) and electronic noise from the electronic components of the system. Although speckle may be useful for tracking tissue motion, often there is a desire to reduce the amount of background noise and speckle in an ultrasound image to increase low-contrast resolution.

Unfortunately, simple averaging is not an effective means for accomplishing speckle reduction in ultrasound because the background speckle signal is highly correlated with the tissue. Temporal compounding (persistence) is the

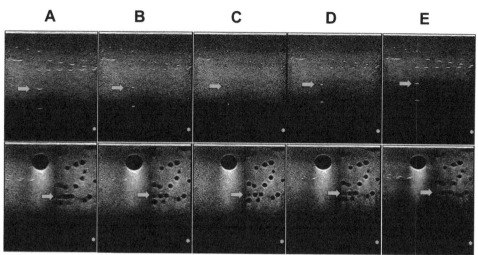

Fig. 2. Speed of sound and phase aberration correction in a phantom. The speed of sound assumed by the scanner was varied to demonstrate the impact on image characteristics of high-contrast targets (*top row*) and anechoic objects (*bottom row*). The speed of sound relative to the phantom (1540 m/s) is F02D120 m/s (*A*), F02D60 m/s (*B*), 0 m/s (*C*), +60 m/s (*D*), and +120 m/s (*E*). Two and other columns (*A, B*) represent object appearances in tissues with lower speeds of sound (such as fatty breasts) whereas two other columns (*D, E*) represent tissue with higher speeds of sound. In all cases, note the loss of lateral resolution (*arrows, top row*), displacement of the target location, and change in the speckle appearance the further away from the true speed of sound (*C*). The percent displacement error is equal to the percent error in the speed of sound estimate. Note the impact on the ability to optimally depict small anechoic objects at depth (*arrows, bottom row*).

traditional approach for reducing speckle in ultrasound. This technique relies on motion or flow between views to decorrelate the speckle and thus reduce the speckle by averaging several frames together. Slight differences between frames due to motion caused by an operator or tissue movement help decorrelate speckle noise, leading to a reduction in speckle.

The speckle pattern is strongly dependent on the center frequency used. With digital broadband beams comes the ability to more easily receive multiple sub-bands at once. Frequency compounding takes multiple frames at different frequencies and averages them together after the detection phase to decorrelate and reduce the speckle signal.[28] Frequency compounding comes with a tradeoff in both penetration and resolution and has diminishing returns when compared with using the full bandwidth as spatial compounding does.[29,30]

Spatial compounding is a technique by which the speckle patterns can be decorrelated by making a composite image with the beam acquired along different paths.[31] Accomplishing this manually and correctly stitching together the images would be extremely difficult and time consuming, which explains why this technique did not emerge commercially until recently. With digitally steered beams and fast signal processing algorithms, spatial compounding has become

a commonly used method for speckle reduction on most modern systems. With spatial compounding, electronic beam steering acquires multiple images[3–13] at different angles followed by registration and reconstruction. The different paths traveled through the tissue lead to a reduction in speckle in the regions where the beam overlaps. Because there is unlikely to be a significant overlap of beams in the extended region of a linear array operating in a trapezoidal acquisition mode, usually the trapezoidal option is disabled during spatial compounding. Spatial compounding techniques are available on virtually all modern ultrasound scanners and go by a variety of trade names (see **Table 1**). Because spatial compounding techniques rely on multiple beam averages, they have an impact on the temporal resolution; however, frame rates can be preserved by using a sliding window correction, which updates with each new view. Additionally, because the images are often composites of beams acquired at multiple angles of insonation, refractive edge and distal shadowing as well as distal enhancement tend to be reduced in these images (**Fig. 4**).

In addition to spatial compounding techniques, many modern systems offer real-time postprocessing techniques for adaptive speckle reduction. These techniques are known by a variety of vendor names (see **Table 1**). In addition to the traditional challenge of trying to filter images

A   **B**

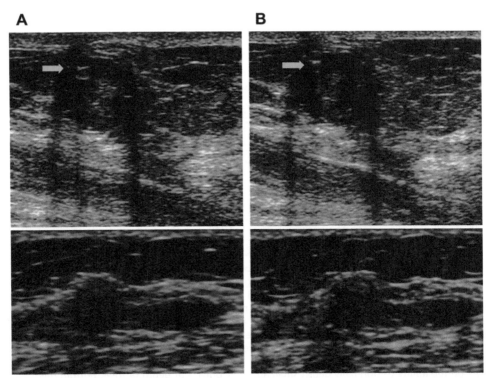

Fig. 3. Speed of sound and phase aberration corrections. (*Top row*) A 66-year-old woman status postlumpectomy presented with an oil cyst without speed of sound correction (*A*) and with speed of sound correction (*B*). Note the change in the presentation of the speckle pattern and the appearance of the high-contrast objects. (*Bottom row*) Sonography in a 44-year-old woman status postmastectomy demonstrates hypoechoic regions consistent with fat necrosis and/or scarring without speed of sound correction (*A*) and with speed of sound correction (*B*). Note the change in the presentation of the speckle pattern and the appearance of the high-contrast objects (*arrows*).

A   **B**   **C**

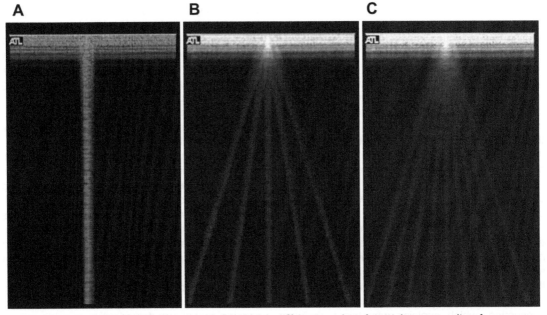

Fig. 4. Depiction of the multiple beams associated with different modes of spatial compounding from an aperture. Shown are normal persistence mode (*A*), 5-beam spatial compounding (*B*), and 9-beam spatial compounding (*C*). In addition to reducing speckle, the combination of multidirectional images tends to blur out distal shadowing and enhancement.

without loss of diagnostic information, ultrasound provides the challenge of having a wealth of structures and noise in the images and a need for the processing to be accomplished in real time. Algorithms aim at analyzing regions for speckle and adaptively removing noise while preserving the echogenic structures in the image, often with some form of edge enhancement to accompany the smoothing process. Because these techniques essentially provide complementary speckle reduction, they are often coupled with spatial compounding to provide a higher degree of speckle reduction when it is desired (**Fig. 5**).[32,33]

Most modern diagnostic ultrasound systems with a breast package feature a combination of spatial compounding and real-time adaptive speckle reduction. Although the literature continues

to evolve as to the benefits and the potential role of these techniques in the breast ultrasound repertoire,[34,35] demand for these options has led to a response in design by several vendors. Regarding future development, even if additional diagnostic information is not garnered for radiologists by these techniques,[36] the noise removal and contrast enhancement are likely to be of value for advancing adjunct technologies, which may benefit by the removal of noise and some distal shadowing artifacts (such as computer-aided diagnosis [CAD] and 3-D reconstruction techniques). Additionally, the appearance of lesions can be affected by the use of one compounding technique versus another, so when findings are presented or reported, it is useful to clarify both the type and the degree of compounding employed as well as

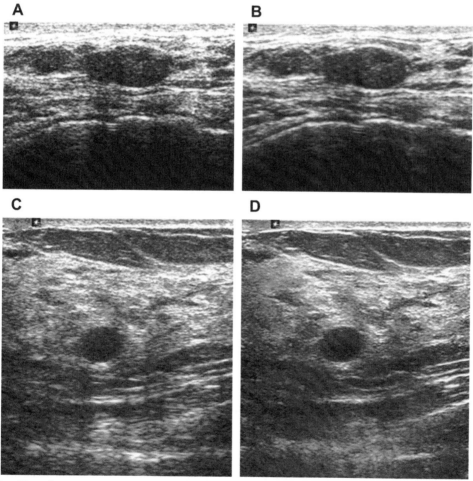

Fig. 5. Speckle reduction technology. A suspected fibroadenoma is shown without spatial compounding (A) and with mild spatial compounding (B). In addition to the change in speckle appearance, note the change in the appearance of specular reflectors in the image as well as the appearance distal to the lesion. A cyst with mild spatial compounding is shown (C) and with higher (13-beam) spatial compounding and real-time speckle reduction (D). Note the dramatic changes in distal features.

whether or not real-time speckle reduction was used.

TISSUE HARMONIC IMAGING

Soft tissue is inherently viscoelastic and, therefore, has an increasingly nonlinear response to ultrasound as the acoustic power is increased. This nonlinear tissue response tends to result in high-pressure (compression) waves traveling faster than low-pressure (rarefaction) waves, which increasingly distorts the wave the further it travels. These distortions shift a portion of the wave energy to harmonic frequencies of the fundamental. Using the broadband nature and digital processing capabilities of modern ultrasound, tissue harmonic imaging (THI) uses signal from the second harmonic (twice the fundamental frequency) of the backscattered echoes as opposed to the fundamental frequency to generate images.[37] For example, for 10-MHz THI, a broadband transducer transmits centered on 5 MHz and receives at 10 MHz. Because the harmonic-generating nonlinear response of the tissue that leads to the received signal is a function of the acoustic power incident on the tissue, echoes returning from the primary lobe of the ultrasound beam are accentuated. The

primary impacts of this effect are to reduce the width of the main lobe and to reduce the amount of side-lobe, grating-lobe, out-of-plane, aberration, and reverberation artifacts in the image (**Fig. 6**).

When used in imaging the breast, THI has been shown to potentially improve contrast between adipose tissue and breast lesions when compared with fundamental frequency images, especially in breasts with mixed adipose and glandular tissue.[38] Additionally, an increase in lesion and acoustic shadow conspicuity as well as definition of lesion borders and internal echoes are potentially improved with THI. Although THI may provide increased contrast in lesions and help clear cysts, it has not been definitively demonstrated to provide any new diagnostic information regarding lesion margins[39] and it does not seem to have an impact on the ability to distinguish benign from malignant lesions at this time.[40]

THI is ubiquitous on modern ultrasound systems, and THI is routinely used in breast ultrasound as an option available for minimizing clutter and clearing internal echoes in cysts. Care must be taken to understand the impact of THI on the displayed image so that mistakes are not made in interpretation. THI technology continues to advance as breast ultrasound transducers

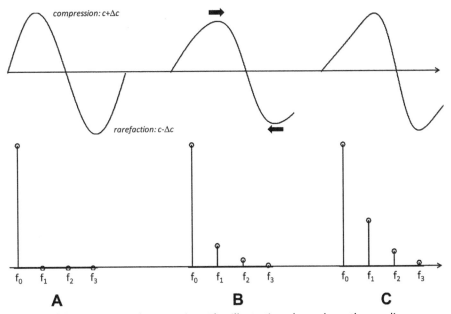

Fig. 6. Illustration of harmonic signal generation. The illustration shows how the nonlinear propagation of a simple sinusoidal waveform (*top row*) gives rise to increasing harmonics of the fundamental frequency (*bottom row*). Increasing harmonics (*along the direction of the arrow*) can be present in detected echoes as a function of increasing propagation depth, increasing tissue nonlinearity parameter (*B/A*), higher incident pressure, higher center frequency, or slower speed of sound. The positive-pressure wave front propagates faster than the negative-pressure wave front, resulting in a sharper transition between compression and rarefaction and an increase in the harmonics of the fundamental frequency present in the spectrum as we move (*A*) to (*C*).

increase in frequency, beamforming is corrected for phase aberration, and different methods for acquiring and processing the harmonic signal are investigated. In particular, methods using the coded pulses (discussed previously) are useful for increasing the quality and penetration of THI, which generally suffer from signal loss due to the reduced energy in the first harmonic. Also, as in harmonic imaging of contrast agents, pulse-inversion subtraction techniques are increasingly used to better suppress the fundamental frequency in the harmonic image to obtain better-quality THI. As THI technology (**Fig. 7**) advances, it would be prudent to periodically review its place in breast ultrasound as an adjunct to fundamental frequency imaging, particularly when THI is used

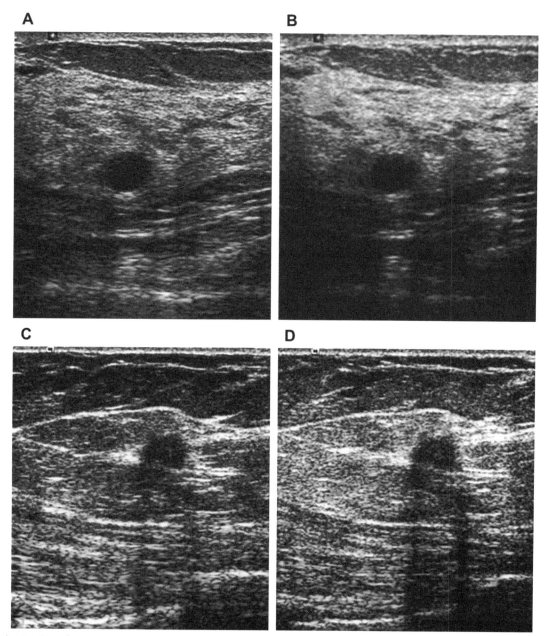

Fig. 7. Tissue harmonic imaging. A cyst with 10-MHz transmit and receive is shown (*A*) and with THI (transmit 5 MHz and receive 10 MHz) (*B*). Below (*C*), (*D*) is an invasive ductal carcinoma at 11.43 MHz transmit and receive (*C*) versus THI (transmit 5 MHz and receive at 10 MHz) (*D*). In both cases, note the change in distal image features and contrast, particularly in the anechoic and the fatty tissue regions.

in conjunction with other image acquisition and processing techniques, such as phase aberration correction and speckle reduction techniques.

DOPPLER ULTRASOUND

The complementary role of Doppler evaluation of suspected lesions is not new to breast ultrasound, and this flow-sensitive technique is useful in evaluating cystic structures, where a finding of flow within the cystic structure is considered a sign of a solid mass. It has been observed that malignant breast lesion vasculature is more conspicuous on Doppler studies than the vasculature of benign lesions.[41] The central components of malignant masses are generally 5 times more vascular than the surrounding fibroglandular tissue. Benign lesions with uniform vasculature are approximately 2 times more vascular than the surrounding tissue.[42] Early clinical investigations found that Doppler imaging corroborated B-mode findings and discovered substantial overlap between malignant and benign lesions.[43,44] Since that time, PD techniques (**Fig. 8**) have essentially replaced color Doppler techniques in breast sonography, because they tend to be more sensitive.

Fully digital modern ultrasound systems and coded excitation should further improve the sensitivity of PD ultrasound. Recent reports seem to indicate that using the currently identified criteria (eg, hypervascularity, vessel penetration, and branching) on 2-D, PD alone has nothing to add in the evaluation of malignant versus benign lesions.[45] 3-D approaches to PD may provide an increase in specificity.[46] These techniques may be aided with the development of CAD techniques.[47] Although still not cleared by the Food and Drug Administration for use in breast imaging, ultrasound contrast agents may be useful for enhancing the ability to identify and quantify vasculature. Ultrasound contrast agents generally use microbubbles, which have a strong harmonic signal due to their nonlinear response and, therefore, may further help in demonstrating vascular lesions. Dynamic contrast harmonic imaging and harmonic PD techniques to visualize the microvasculature and evaluate contrast kinetics continue to be an active area of developing research.[48–50]

IMAGING TISSUE ELASTICITY

One of the main components of a clinical breast examination is palpation. Solid breast masses tend to be more resistive to changes in their shape than the surrounding glandular and fatty tissues that make up the breast. The amount of resulting tissue motion (strain) induced by an applied pressure (stress) is an approximate constant (modulus) of the tissue and the boundary conditions. Elastography is an ultrasound imaging technique, which attempts to perform a sort of palpation by generating maps that reflect this modulus. Generally, there is a tendency for cysts to not be as hard as the background fibroglandular parenchyma and for solid masses to be harder, with malignant masses and lymph nodes tending to be harder than benign masses, such as fibroadenomas.[51] This potential for elastography to provide additional information to improve the specificity of ultrasound in the breast was a primary drive for the initial applications of the technique.[52,53] Several vendors have released their first-generation elastography packages. All require light compression applied to the breast in the longitudinal direction of the beam. In most cases, the resulting tissue deformation is estimated from the ultrasound data and displayed as an estimate of the tissue longitudinal strain (static elastography). This approach is user dependent and nonquantitative. Initial clinical studies investigating breast ultrasound elastography integrated the BI-RADS ultrasound lexicon[3,4] into the studies and showed potential for the technique but failed to demonstrate any consistent benefit to B-mode

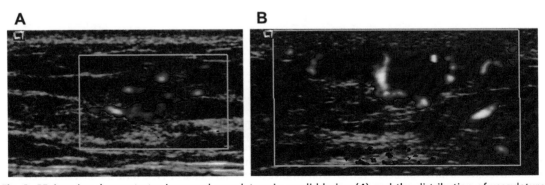

Fig. 8. PD imaging demonstrates increased vasculature in a solid lesion (A) and the distribution of vasculature around a cyst (B).

ultrasound by elastography.[54,55] More recent studies indicate that there might be a potential increase in specificity for certain types of lesions when coupled with conventional B-mode ultrasound[56,57] but problems relating to reproducibility remain.

A new generation of ultrasound elastography technology is emerging that does not rely on highly user-dependent, free-hand compression techniques to obtain static longitudinal strain estimates. These new techniques use the acoustic radiation field generated by the transducer itself to remotely deliver an impulse to the tissue.[58,59] The subtle ultrasound-induced tissue motion can be detected by the transducer, and strain images are generated that do not rely on user compression.

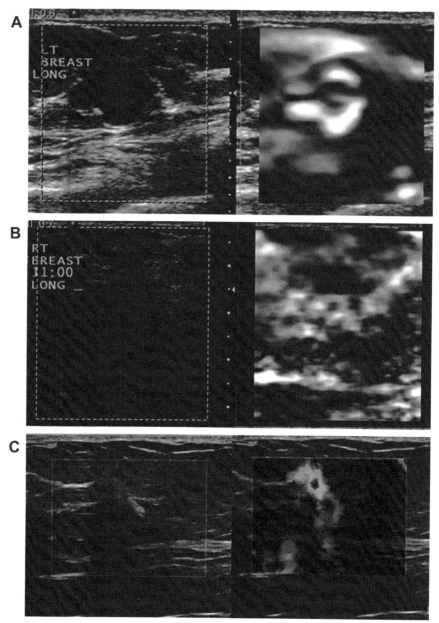

Fig. 9. Elastographic imaging. Top row (*A*) shows the B-mode image (*left*) and accompanying static elastogram (*right*) for a cyst demonstrating the typical bull's eye appearance of low hardness surrounding artifact whereas middle row (*B*) demonstrates the harder appearance of invasive ductal carcinoma. Bottom row (*C*) shows a hard invasive ductal carcinoma imaged using nonstatic shear wave elastography (*red* represents hard tissue and *blue* represents soft tissue).

These impulses generate shear waves. A specific anatomic location can be scanned rapidly to facilitate estimation of the shear wave velocity and, therefore, produce a quantitative measure of elasticity. These emerging techniques rely on extremely fast imaging and processing techniques as well as slight transducer modifications, and they have the potential to address the problem of user dependence, with fewer artifacts from boundary conditions and with a more quantitative approach. Because this seems the most promising approach to reliable ultrasound elastography (**Fig. 9**), several vendors have implemented this technology.

COMPUTER-AIDED DIAGNOSIS

As with mammography, there is mounting evidence that consistent use of a standardized lexicon may lead to higher sensitivity and specificity in the diagnosis of ultrasound lesions. BI-RADS of breast ultrasound features is increasing.[60,61] Standardized reporting of features is amenable to computer-aided approaches for detection and diagnosis. Additionally, as with MRI evaluation of the breast, as multiple contrast mechanisms and 3-D acquisitions of breast ultrasound mature, there is likely to be a move toward increased dependence on breast ultrasound CAD applications. Breast ultrasound CAD may aid in visualization, evaluation, and standardized reporting of breast ultrasound examinations,[62–64] particularly as increasingly larger volumes are collected for screening studies.[65] As with the rest of the emerging and maturing technology (described previously), substantial research is needed to identify the potential and the limitations of CAD in breast ultrasound.

SUMMARY

A decade into the paradigm shift of digital ultrasound, technology continues to evolve rapidly, and new technology is being introduced into the clinic at an astounding pace. Advances in acquisition techniques to help increase the penetration, contrast, and resolution of breast ultrasound have been fueled by the move to fully digital broadband systems with dedicated signal processing boards for beamforming, reconstruction, and image postprocessing. Many of these systems and techniques are in their second or higher generations. Many of these technologies come with associated imaging artifacts that may alter the appearance of traditional imaging markers used for diagnosis. In the adoption of these new imaging techniques, which can have a great impact on image interpretation, care

should be taken in how and when this technology is applied. These considerations may have an impact on the time needed to interpret an ultrasound examination as well as the time to acquire the necessary data for the examination.

Another immediate consequence for workflow in clinics is that system presets are more important than ever. Despite an increase in automated optimization, there is an increasing number of options that are often too difficult and time consuming to optimize in real time. Many features should only be used under certain circumstances. Additionally, the use of EFV, digital cine, and 3-D/4-D methods means that ultrasound systems will require more storage space on picture archiving and communication systems.

With steadily increasing image quality and many new and maturing contrast mechanisms, ultrasound seems poised to advance its position in the clinical evaluation of breast lesions by revealing nonpalpable, mammographically occult carcinomas and multifocal and multicentric disease. The clinical research performed should investigate the new techniques and assess how the new techniques are integrated. In addition, research should aim to determine which patients are most likely to benefit from a technology or a combination of technologies. With all the potential combinations available, carefully controlled, quantitative clinical feasibility research and analysis are needed.

ACKNOWLEDGMENTS

We thank Barbara Almarez Mahinda for assistance in manuscript preparation.

REFERENCES

1. Thompson M, Klimberg VS. Use of ultrasound in breast surgery. Surg Clin North Am 2007;87(2):469–84.
2. Yang W, Dempsey PJ. Diagnostic breast ultrasound: current status and future directions. Radiol Clin North Am 2007;45(5):845–61.
3. Mendelson E, Berg W, Merritt C. Toward a standardized breast ultrasound lexicon, BI-RADS: ultrasound+. Semin Roentgenol 2001;36:217–25.
4. American College of Radiology (ACR). ACR BI-RADS—ultrasound. In: Breast imaging reporting and data system, breast imaging Atlas. Reston (VA): American College of Radiology; 2003. p.117.
5. Nothacker M, Duda V, Hahn M, et al. Early detection of breast cancer: benefits and risks of supplemental breast ultrasound in asymptomatic women with mammographically dense breast tissue. A systematic review. BMC Cancer 2009;9:335.

6. Greene T, Cocilovo C, Estabrook A, et al. A single institution review of new breast malignancies identified solely by sonography. J Am Coll Surg 2006; 203(6):894–8.

7. Berg WA, Blume JD, Cormack JB, et al. Combined screening with ultrasound and mammography vs mammography alone in women at elevated risk of breast cancer. JAMA 2008;299(18):2151–63.

8. Forsberg F. Ultrasonic biomedical technology; marketing versus clinical reality. Ultrasonics 2004; 42(1–9):17–27.

9. Whittingham TA. An overview of digital technology in ultrasonic imaging. Eur Radiol 1999;9(Suppl 3): S307–11.

10. Pedersen MH, Misaridis TX, Jensen JA. Clinical evaluation of chirp-coded excitation in medical ultrasound. Ultrasound Med Biol 2003;29(6):895–905.

11. Misaridis T, Jensen JA. Use of modulated excitation signals in medical ultrasound. Part I: basic concepts and expected benefits. IEEE Trans Ultrason Ferroelectr Freq Control 2005;52(2):177–91.

12. Chiao RY, Hao XH. Coded excitation for diagnostic ultrasound: a system developer's perspective. IEEE Trans Ultrason Ferroelectr Freq Control 2005;52(2): 160–70.

13. Harvey CJ, Pilcher JM, Eckersley RJ, et al. Advances in ultrasound. Clin Radiol 2002;57(3):157–77.

14. Claudon M, Tranquart F, Evans DH, et al. Advances in ultrasound. Eur Radiol 2002;12(1):7–18.

15. Whittingham TA. Broadband transducers. Eur Radiol 1999;9(Suppl 3):S298–303.

16. Rizzatto G. Evolution of ultrasound transducers: 1.5 and 2D arrays. Eur Radiol 1999;9(Suppl 3): S304–6.

17. Hanafy A. Broadband phased array transducer design with frequency-controlled two-dimensional capability. Ultrasonic Transducer Engineering 1998;3341: 64–82. Available at: http://full_record.do?product= UA&search_mode=GeneralSearch&qid=3&SID= 1F2hC2DgPFmDkjmDHGe&page=1&doc=1& colname=WOS. Accessed February 17, 2011.

18. Weng L, Tirumalai AP, Lowery CM, et al. US extended-field-of-view imaging technology. Radiology 1997; 203(3):877–80.

19. Fornage BD, Atkinson EN, Nock LF, et al. US with extended field of view: phantom-tested accuracy of distance measurements. Radiology 2000;214(2): 579–84.

20. Kotsianos-Hermle D, Wirth S, Fischer T, et al. First clinical use of a standardized three-dimensional ultrasound for breast imaging. Eur J Radiol 2009; 71(1):102–8.

21. Scanlan KA. Sonographic artifacts and their origins. AJR Am J Roentgenol 1991;156(6):1267–72.

22. O'Donnell M, Flax SW. Phase aberration measurements in medical ultrasound: human studies. Ultrason Imaging 1988;10(1):1–11.

23. Trahey GE, Freiburger PD, Nock LF, et al. In vivo measurements of ultrasonic beam distortion in the breast. Ultrason Imaging 1991;13(1):71–90.

24. Trahey GE, Smith SW. Properties of acoustical speckle in the presence of phase aberration. Part I: first order statistics. Ultrason Imaging 1988;10(1):12–28.

25. Barr RG, Rim A, Graham R, et al. Speed of sound imaging: improved image quality in breast sonography. Ultrasound Q 2009;25(3):141–4.

26. Anderson ME, McKeag MS, Trahey GE. The impact of sound speed errors on medical ultrasound imaging. J Acoust Soc Am 2000;107(6):3540–8.

27. Burckhardt CB. Speckle in ultrasound B-mode scans. IEEE Transactions on Sonics and Ultrasonics 1978; 25(1):1–6. Available at: http://full_record.do?product= UA&search_mode=GeneralSearch&qid=5&SID= 1F2hC2DgPFmDkjmDHGe&page=1&doc=2&colname= WOS. Accessed February 17, 2011.

28. Magnin PA, von Ramm OT, Thurstone FL. Frequency compounding for speckle contrast reduction in phased array images. Ultrason Imaging 1982;4(3): 267–81.

29. Trahey GE, Allison JW, Smith SW, et al. A quantitative approach to speckle reduction via frequency compounding. Ultrason Imaging 1986;8(3):151–64.

30. Wagner RF, Insana MF, Smith SW. Fundamental correlation lengths of coherent speckle in medical ultrasonic images. IEEE Trans Ultrason Ferroelectr Freq Control 1988;35(1):34–44.

31. Trahey GE, Smith SW, von Ramm OT. Speckle pattern correlation with lateral aperture translation: experimental results and implications for spatial compounding. IEEE Trans Ultrason Ferroelectr Freq Control 1986;33(3):257–64.

32. Meuwly JY, Thiran JP, Gudinchet F. Application of adaptive image processing technique to real-time spatial compound ultrasound imaging improves image quality. Invest Radiol 2003;38(5):257–62.

33. Barr RG, Maldonado RL, Georgian-Smith D. Comparison of conventional, compounding, computer enhancement, and compounding with computer enhancement in ultrasound imaging of the breast. Ultrasound Q 2009;25(3):129–34.

34. Huber S, Wagner M, Medl M, et al. Real-time spatial compound imaging in breast ultrasound. Ultrasound Med Biol 2002;28(2):155–63.

35. Kwak JY, Kim EK, You JK, et al. Variable breast conditions: comparison of conventional and real-time compound ultrasonography. J Ultrasound Med 2004;23(1):85–96.

36. Cha JH, Moon WK, Cho N, et al. Differentiation of benign from malignant solid breast masses: conventional US versus spatial compound imaging. Radiology 2005;237(3):841–6.

37. Tranquart F, Grenier N, Eder V, et al. Clinical use of ultrasound tissue harmonic imaging. Ultrasound Med Biol 1999;25(6):889–94.

38. Szopinski KT, Pajk AM, Wysocki M, et al. Tissue harmonic imaging: utility in breast sonography. J Ultrasound Med 2003;22(5):479–87 [quiz: 488–9].

39. Rosen EL, Soo MS. Tissue harmonic imaging sonography of breast lesions: improved margin analysis, conspicuity, and image quality compared to conventional ultrasound. Clin Imaging 2001;25(6):379–84.

40. Cha JH, Moon WK, Cho N, et al. Characterization of benign and malignant solid breast masses: comparison of conventional US and tissue harmonic imaging. Radiology 2007;242(1):63–9.

41. Cosgrove DO, Kedar RP, Bamber JC, et al. Breast diseases: color Doppler US in differential diagnosis. Radiology 1993;189(1):99–104.

42. Sehgal CM, Arger PH, Rowling SE, et al. Quantitative vascularity of breast masses by Doppler imaging: regional variations and diagnostic implications. J Ultrasound Med 2000;19(7):427–40 [quiz: 441–2].

43. Ozdemir A, Ozdemir H, Maral I, et al. Differential diagnosis of solid breast lesions: contribution of Doppler studies to mammography and gray scale imaging. J Ultrasound Med 2001;20(10):1091–101.

44. Buadu LD, Murakami J, Murayama S, et al. Colour Doppler sonography of breast masses: a multiparameter analysis. Clin Radiol 1997;52(12):917–23.

45. Gokalp G, Topal U, Kizilkaya E. Power Doppler sonography: anything to add to BI-RADS US in solid breast masses? Eur J Radiol 2009;70(1):77–85.

46. LeCarpentier GL, Roubidoux MA, Fowlkes JB, et al. Suspicious breast lesions: assessment of 3D Doppler US indexes for classification in a test population and fourfold cross-validation scheme. Radiology 2008;249(2):463–70.

47. Huang YL, Kuo SJ, Hsu CC, et al. Computer-aided diagnosis for breast tumors by using vascularization of 3-D power Doppler ultrasound. Ultrasound Med Biol 2009;35(10):1607–14.

48. Moon WK, Im JG, Noh DY, et al. Nonpalpable breast lesions: evaluation with power Doppler US and a microbubble contrast agent-initial experience. Radiology 2000;217(1):240–6.

49. Clevert D, Jung EM, Jungius KP, et al. Value of tissue harmonic imaging (THI) and contrast harmonic imaging (CHI) in detection and characterisation of breast tumours. Eur Radiol 2007;17(1):1–10.

50. Kettenbach J, Helbich TH, Huber S, et al. Computer-assisted quantitative assessment of power Doppler US: effects of microbubble contrast agent in the differentiation of breast tumors. Eur J Radiol 2005;53(2):238–44.

51. Sewell CW. Pathology of benign and malignant breast disorders. Radiol Clin North Am 1995;33(6):1067–80.

52. Cespedes I, Ophir J, Ponnekanti H, et al. Elastography: elasticity imaging using ultrasound with application to muscle and breast in vivo. Ultrason Imaging 1993;15(2):73–88.

53. Garra BS, Cespedes EI, Ophir J, et al. Elastography of breast lesions: initial clinical results. Radiology 1997;202(1):79–86.

54. Itoh A, Ueno E, Tohno E, et al. Breast disease: clinical application of US elastography for diagnosis. Radiology 2006;239(2):341–50.

55. Thomas A, Kummel S, Fritzsche F, et al. Real-time sonoelastography performed in addition to B-mode ultrasound and mammography: improved differentiation of breast lesions? Acad Radiol 2006;13(12):1496–504.

56. Burnside ES, Hall TJ, Sommer AM, et al. Differentiating benign from malignant solid breast masses with US strain imaging. Radiology 2007;245(2):401–10.

57. Scaperrotta G, Ferranti C, Costa C, et al. Role of sonoelastography in non-palpable breast lesions. Eur Radiol 2008;18(11):2381–9.

58. Athanasiou A, Tardivon A, Tanter M, et al. Breast lesions: quantitative elastography with supersonic shear imaging–preliminary results. Radiology 2010;256(1):297–303.

59. Garra BS. Imaging and estimation of tissue elasticity by ultrasound. Ultrasound Q 2007;23(4):255–68.

60. Costantini M, Belli P, Lombardi R, et al. Characterization of solid breast masses: use of the sonographic breast imaging reporting and data system lexicon. J Ultrasound Med 2006;25(5):649–59 [quiz: 661].

61. Kim EK, Ko KH, Oh KK, et al. Clinical application of the BI-RADS final assessment to breast sonography in conjunction with mammography. AJR Am J Roentgenol 2008;190(5):1209–15.

62. Shen WC, Chang RF, Moon WK, et al. Breast ultrasound computer-aided diagnosis using BI-RADS features. Acad Radiol 2007;14(8):928–39.

63. Drukker K, Gruszauskas NP, Sennett CA, et al. Breast US computer-aided diagnosis workstation: performance with a large clinical diagnostic population. Radiology 2008;248(2):392–7.

64. Gruszauskas NP, Drukker K, Giger ML, et al. Breast US computer-aided diagnosis system: robustness across urban populations in South Korea and the United States. Radiology 2009;253(3):661–71.

65. Sahiner B, Chan HP, Roubidoux MA, et al. Malignant and benign breast masses on 3D US volumetric images: effect of computer-aided diagnosis on radiologist accuracy. Radiology 2007;242(3):716–24.

Ultrasound of Invasive Lobular Carcinoma

Margaret Adejolu, MRCP, FRCR[a,b],
Savitri Krishnamurthy, MD[c], Gary J. Whitman, MD[d,*]

KEYWORDS

• Ultrasound • Invasive lobular carcinoma • Breast cancer

Invasive lobular carcinoma (ILC) was first described as a distinct histologic type of breast cancer by Foote and Stewart in 1946.[1] ILC is the second most common type of breast malignancy after invasive ductal carcinoma (IDC) and constitutes about 4% to 15% of all breast cancers.[2–4] ILC is notoriously difficult to detect clinically and mammographically because of its incohesive histologic growth pattern, absence of a strong desmoplastic reaction, low likelihood of producing calcifications, and low mammographic density.[5,6] This article reviews the histopathological and the imaging appearances of ILC, with particular emphasis on the appearance of ILC on sonography.

EPIDEMIOLOGY

In 2009, the Centers for Disease Control and Prevention (CDC) published the results of a population-based analysis of data on in situ and invasive lobular and ductal breast cancer from 44 states and the District of Columbia for the years 1999 to 2004. These data were representative of 92.1% of the US population and were obtained from 2 cancer registries, the National Program of Cancer Registries (NPCR) and the Surveillance, Epidemiology and End Results (SEER) program of the National Cancer Institute. The results, which were published by Eheman and colleagues,[4]

showed that the incidence rate of ILC was 10.6 cases per 100,000 women, compared with 86.3 cases of IDC per 100,000 women. Eheman and colleagues found that the incidence rates for ILC increased with age, peaking among women aged 70 to 79 years, and declining slightly at 80 years of age. The rates of IDC also increased steadily up to age 79 years. There was a steep increase in IDC rates among women in the 40- to 49-year age group, which was not evident in the ILC population. Eheman and colleagues[4] also analyzed the age-standardized incidence rates of invasive lobular and ductal breast cancers for race and ethnicity and found that the incidence rates for both groups were highest among Caucasian women, while Asian/Pacific Islander women had the lowest rates.

Eheman and colleagues[4] also found that the incidence rates for invasive lobular and mixed lobular-ductal breast cancers decreased from 1999 to 2004, while the incidence of IDC decreased from 2000 to 2003 and plateaued in 2004. In contrast, Li and colleagues,[7] in an earlier but smaller study, found that the incidence rates of ILC increased steadily while the incidence rates of IDC remained essentially constant over the period from 1987 to 1999. There is some evidence that the decrease in the incidence of ILC in recent years is associated with a decrease in hormone therapy use, as lobular carcinomas are more

[a] Department of Radiology, King's College Hospital, Denmark Hill, London SE5 9RS, UK
[b] Department of Diagnostic Radiology, The University of Texas MD Anderson Cancer Center, 1515 Holcombe Boulevard, Houston, TX 77030, USA
[c] Department of Pathology, The University of Texas MD Anderson Cancer Center, 1515 Holcombe Boulevard, Houston, TX 77030, USA
[d] Departments of Diagnostic Radiology and Radiation Oncology, The University of Texas MD Anderson Cancer Center, Unit 1350, PO Box 301439, Houston TX 77230-1439, USA
* Corresponding author. Departments of Diagnostic Radiology and Radiation Oncology, The University of Texas MD Anderson Cancer Center, Unit 1350, PO Box 301439, Houston TX 77230-1439.
E-mail address: gwhitman@mdanderson.org

Ultrasound Clin 6 (2011) 313–325
doi:10.1016/j.cult.2011.04.002
1556-858X/11/$ – see front matter © 2011 Elsevier Inc. All rights reserved.

sensitive to the effects of hormone therapy than ductal carcinomas.[7,8]

PATHOLOGY

On gross pathologic inspection, ILC typically forms a hard mass with irregular borders. In some cases, there may be no distinct mass but rather a subtle, diffuse indurated area.[9] Histologically, ILC is composed of loosely cohesive small round cells that invade the surrounding tissue in single files or small clusters. The lack of cohesion exhibited by these cells is thought to be due to lack of expression of E-cadherin, a transmembrane glycoprotein involved in epithelial cell-to-cell adhesion. Previous studies have demonstrated complete loss of E-cadherin expression in 80% to 100% of ILC cases.[10]

ILC may be classified into several histologic subtypes based on the predominant morphologic pattern. The predominant subtype, classic ILC, is characterized by noncohesive cells arranged in single cell rows, forming linear cords. This cellular arrangement has been called the Indian file pattern (**Fig. 1**). These single rows of cells may form concentric arrays around ductules and lobules, resulting in a targetoid pattern.[9,10] Orvieto and colleagues,[11] in a study of 530 cases of pure ILC, found that 57% of the cases were classic ILC. Classic ILC is the subtype most commonly associated with lobular carcinoma in situ (LCIS), and coexistent LCIS is found in 90% of cases of classic ILC.[12]

Nonclassic ILC consists of several subtypes. In alveolar ILC, tumor cells similar to those seen in the classic type are clustered in aggregates of greater than 20 cells, separated by thin bands of fibrous stroma.[10] In solid ILC, tumor cells diffusely infiltrate the surrounding tissues in large solid sheets, with little intervening stroma.[10] The signet ring subtype is composed of signet cells characterized by intracytoplasmic accumulation of mucin. Signet cells may be present as components of other subtypes (**Fig. 2**).[9] The tubulo–lobular variant of ILC is characterized by an infiltrative pattern similar to that of classic ILC, with some tumor cells organized in tubular structures.[10] In pleomorphic ILC, the distinctive growth pattern is similar to that seen in the classic type, but the neoplastic cells demonstrate marked cellular pleomorphism and nuclear atypia.[10] Pleomorphic ILC may show apocrine or histiocytoid differentiation. Mixed forms, consisting of different subtypes of ILC, may occur, usually with classic ILC in combination with other subtypes.[10]

The pleomorphic subtype is considered to be a particularly aggressive subtype of ILC because of its peculiar histopathologic and biologic characteristics which include more pronounced cytologic changes, a higher rate of peritumoral vascular invasion, a lower rate of expression of hormone receptors, and a higher rate of overexpression/amplification of the HER-2/neu gene when compared with other subtypes.[11,13] Tumors cells in ILC are usually estrogen receptor (ER) and progesterone receptor (PR) positive, without overexpression or amplification of the HER-2/neu gene. Orvieto and colleagues[11] reported ER and/or PR positivity in 93.6% of the 530 ILCs in their study.

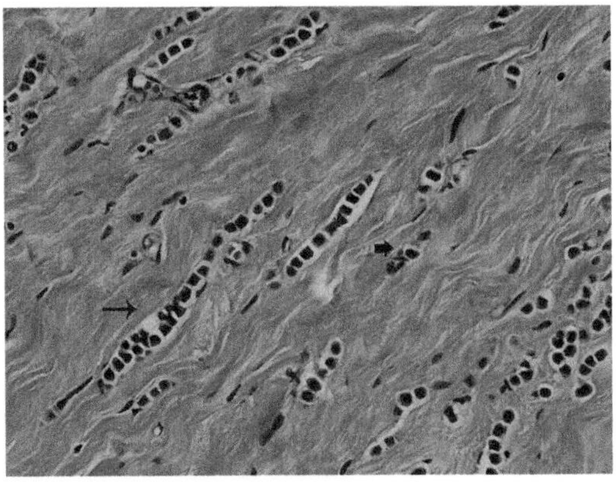

Fig. 1. Photomicrograph shows classic invasive lobular carcinoma (ILC) with low nuclear grade tumor cells arranged singly (*short arrow*) and in linear strands (*long arrow*) in a background of dense fibrosis (hematoxylin–eosin, original magnification × 20). (*From* Whitman GJ, Huynh PT, Patel P, et al. Sonography of invasive lobular carcinoma. Ultrasound Clin 2007;1:656; with permission.)

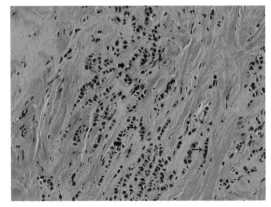

Fig. 2. Photomicrograph shows evidence of invasive lobular carcinoma (ILC) with discohesive tumor cells of intermediate grade arranged predominantly in linear cords (*long arrows*), with a few scattered signet ring cells (*short arrows*) (hematoxylin–eosin, original magnification × 20). (*From* Whitman GJ, Huynh PT, Patel P, et al. Sonography of invasive lobular carcinoma. Ultrasound Clin 2007;1:650; with permission.)

CLINICAL FEATURES

The most common clinical presentation of ILC is that of an ill-defined mass. ILC often fails to form discrete, readily palpable masses as a consequence of its discohesive cellular pattern and relative paucity of desmoplastic stromal alteration. In these cases, a subtle diffuse area of thickening or skin retraction may be the only clinical abnormality.[9,10]

ILC may spread via lymphatic or hematogeneous dissemination. There is a higher incidence of metastases to bone in ILC when compared with IDC. ILC is less likely than IDC to metastasize to the lungs, the pleura, the liver, and the brain.[14,15] ILC has a predilection for spread to the peritoneal (**Fig. 3**) and leptomeningeal surfaces, the gastrointestinal tract and the ovaries.[14–16] It is thought that the loss of adhesiveness of tumor cells as a result of loss of expression of the cell–cell adhesion molecule E-cadherin in ILC facilitates this form of metastases and also plays a role in the increased propensity for bilateral tumors and the multifocal and multicentric distribution of disease often seen in ILC.[14]

MAMMOGRAPHIC FEATURES

ILC may be difficult to detect on mammography, as it often presents with very subtle features (**Fig. 4**) and may be mammographically occult. The reported false negative rates for the detection of ILC on mammography are higher than other histological types of breast cancers. False-negative rates of up to 19% have been reported for ILC.[3] The sensitivity of mammography for detecting ILC has been reported to range between 57% and 79%.[6,17]

The relatively low sensitivity of mammography for the detection of ILC compared with other types of breast cancers is due to a combination of factors. ILC's tendency to infiltrate into the surrounding stroma in rows of single cells, with little disruption of the underlying tissues, makes it less likely than other types of cancers to form discrete masses. Subtle mammographic features, such as asymmetric densities and architectural distortions, tend to be more common in ILC than in IDC.[14] The mammographic diagnosis of ILC is also limited by the fact that the density of ILC on mammography is similar to, or less than that of normal glandular tissue, due to the noncohesive

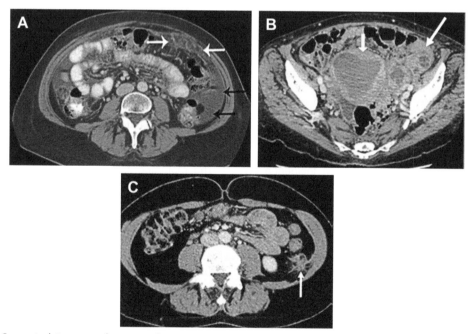

Fig. 3. Computed tomography scans demonstrate peritoneal and omental metastatic disease from invasive lobular carcinoma (ILC). (*A*) Thickening of the greater omentum (*white arrows*) due to metastatic disease. A moderate amount of ascites is noted (*black arrows.*) (*B*) Mural thickening of small bowel loops (*long arrow*) is noted within the pelvis, along with irregular bladder wall thickening (*short arrow*) due to metastatic disease. This patient later developed small bowel obstruction. (*C*) There is an enhancing spiculated metastatic deposit (*arrow*) in the large bowel mesentery. (*From* Whitman GJ, Huynh PT, Patel P, et al. Sonography of invasive lobular carcinoma. Ultrasound Clin 2007;1:647; with permission.)

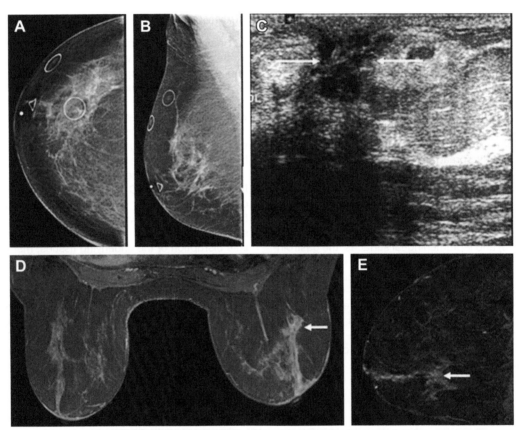

Fig. 4. The patient presented with a palpable abnormality in the retroareolar aspect of the right breast. A radi-opaque marker was placed on the nipple, and round markers were placed on skin lesions. Craniocaudal (*A*) and mediolateral oblique mammograms (*B*) show no abnormalities besides nipple retraction in the region of the palpable abnormality (indicated by the *triangular marker*). (*C*) Sonography in the region of the palpable abnor-mality shows an irregular hypoechoic mass (*arrows*) with posterior shadowing. Ultrasound-guided core needle biopsy of the mass revealed invasive lobular carcinoma (ILC). (*D*) Axial postcontrast magnetic resonance imaging (MRI) demonstrates an enhancing mass (*arrow*), with enhancement extending from the nipple to the mass. (*E*) Sagittal subtraction image shows the mass (*arrow*) and irregular enhancement extending to the nipple in a linear distribution. MRI-guided core biopsy of the mass revealed ILC. Mastectomy was performed, and the extent of disease correlated well with the enhancing findings noted on MRI.

nature of the ILC cells.[18] The low incidence of associated microcalcifications is another cause for the reduced sensitivity of mammography for the detection of ILC. In a study of 6009 cancers, Le Gal and colleagues[17] found suspicious micro-calcification in 24% of the cases of pure ILC, in 32% of the cases of mixed ILC and IDC, and in 41% of the cases of other cancers, a group con-sisting mainly of IDCs.

The use of computer-aided detection (CAD) in mammography has been shown to significantly improve the sensitivity of mammography for the detection of ILC. Evans and colleagues[19] reported a sensitivity of 91% (86 of 94 ILCs) when CAD was applied to digitized films. The and colleagues[20] reported a sensitivity of 100% when CAD was applied to full-field digital mammography images to identify 7 out of 7 ILCs.

The mammographic appearances of ILC are variable. Discrete masses with spiculated, poorly defined, or well-defined margins are the most common appearances (**Fig. 5**). The study of 6,009 cases of breast cancers by Le Gal and colleagues included 455 (7.6%) cases of ILC. This comprised of 341 (75%) cases of pure ILC and 114 (25%) ILC mixed with ductal forms.[17]

Le Gal and colleagues compared the mammo-graphic features of the ILC cases with other types of breast cancer. They found that ILC was less likely to present as a mass than other histological subtypes (51% compared with 63%). They also found that pure ILCs were less frequently round in shape (1% compared with 11%) and were more likely to have spiculated margins (28% compared with 23%) or present as architectural distortions on mammography (18% compared

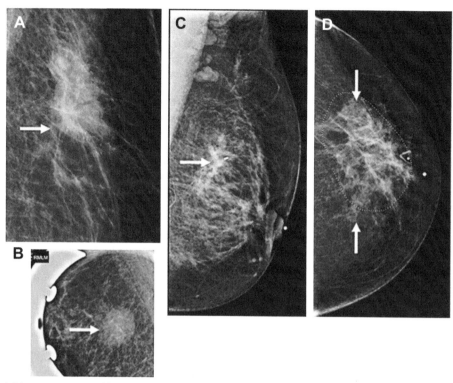

Fig. 5. Variable appearances of invasive lobular carcinoma (ILC) on mammography. (*A*) Mediolateral oblique view shows an irregular mass with indistinct margins and associated pleomorphic microcalcifications (*arrow*). (*B*) Magnified lateromedial view shows a well-defined, oval mass with circumscribed margins (*arrow*). (*C*) Mediolateral oblique mammogram shows an area of architectural distortion (*arrow*) and an associated clip marker. (*D*) Craniocaudal mammogram shows a large area of architectural distortion (*arrows* and outlined area) in the region of the palpable abnormality (noted by the *triangular marker*).

with 6%) when compared with other histological subtypes of breast carcinoma. It is noteworthy that architectural distortions, which are often regarded as subtle mammographic abnormalities that can be easily missed, were 3 times more common in ILC than in IDC.

Hilleren and colleagues[21] conducted a study on the mammographic appearances of 185 cases of ILC and found spiculated masses in 53% of the cases, architectural distortions in 16%, poorly defined opacities in 7%, normal or benign findings in 16%, and parenchymal asymmetries in 4% of the cases. Le Gal and colleagues suggested that the disparity in the proportion of spiculated masses in the studies by Hilleren and colleagues and by Le Gal and colleagues[17] was a consequence of differences in the criteria used in describing a mass as spiculated. Le Gal and colleagues concluded that a proportion of the masses described by Hilleren and colleagues as spiculated masses would have been classified as poorly defined masses by their criteria.[17,21]

Garnett and colleagues[22] studied the mammographic features of 59 cases of ILC and 59 cases of IDC and found that ILCs were seen more

distinctly on the craniocaudal (CC) views, where they were more likely to present as a spiculated masses, compared with vague regions of architectural distortion or asymmetries on the mediolateral oblique (MLO) views. IDCs were seen equally well on both the CC and the MLO views. Garnett and colleagues[22] also found that IDCs were usually isolated from the parenchymal density, while the ILCs were usually found within, or on the edge of, the parenchymal density. Hilleren and colleagues[21] additionally found that subtle mammographic signs such as architectural distortions were seen with greater frequency on the CC views compared with the MLO and the lateral views.

Another mammographic feature of ILC is a decrease in breast size. Harvey and colleagues retrospectively reviewed serial mammograms in 30 ILC patients and identified ipsilateral reduction in breast size in 5 of the 30 patients. Harvey and colleagues described this finding as a late indicator of ILC, mainly seen when the tumor burden is large. The authors attributed this finding to decreased compressibility of the breast, resulting from tumor infiltration. Harvey and colleagues[23] also showed that that ipsilateral reduction in breast size was commonly associated with a clinically palpable area of breast thickening and was more likely to be associated with an asymmetric density or a region of architectural distortion than a discrete mass on mammography.

Jafri and colleagues[24] described a similar but more subtle mammographic feature of ILC. Jafri and colleagues[24] reported 2 cases of ILC with an apparent decrease in the breast glandular tissue volume with preservation of the mammographic breast size, when the current mammograms were compared with previous ones. Jafri and colleagues reported that this finding occurred earlier than the generalized decrease in breast size as described by Harvey and colleagues.[23,24] The finding described by Jafri and colleagues[24] is thought to be due to malignant infiltration of the glandular tissues.

ULTRASOUND APPEARANCES

Ultrasound is an important adjunct to mammography and clinical examination in the evaluation of breast lesions. Ultrasound has an established role in determining if a clinically or mammographically apparent lesion is real or artifactual, and helps to further characterize lesions by differentiating solid from cystic lesions. Ultrasound also provides guidance for interventional procedures performed in breast imaging such as biopsies, aspirations, drainages, and needle localizations.

The sensitivity of ultrasound for the detection of ILC is greater than that of mammography, with sensitivities ranging from 68% to 98%.[25–28] The use of ultrasound as an adjunct to mammography has been shown to significantly improve the detection of ILC. Butler and colleagues reviewed 81 mammographically subtle or invisible lesions and found that 87.7% (71 of 81) of the lesions were readily detectable on sonography. Butler and colleagues[28] also reported sonographic abnormalities in 73.3% (11 of 15) of cases with suspicious clinical findings and negative mammograms.

Ultrasound has been shown to provide a more accurate measurement of the size of a mass than mammography or clinical examination. Berg and colleagues[29] found that ultrasound provided a more accurate measurement of the size of a mass compared with mammography, and the findings on ultrasound resulted in a change in surgical management in 18% of the patients. Ultrasound is superior to mammography in identifying multicentricity and multifocality, and sonography is therefore particularly useful in the work-up of patients with ILC (**Fig. 6**).

Berg and colleagues,[29] in a study of 40 patients with mixed histologic types of breast cancer, found that, using pathologic specimens as the gold standard, ultrasound demonstrated 94% (45/48) of invasive tumor foci and 44% (7 of 16) of foci of ductal carcinoma in situ (DCIS). Mammography demonstrated 81% (39 of 48) of invasive tumor foci and 88% (14 of 16) foci of DCIS. Nine of 64 (14%) malignant foci were only seen on sonography. Fifteen percent (3 of 20) of the patients suspected of having unifocal disease on mammography required wider excision, based on the ultrasound findings.

Moon and colleagues[30] found clinically and mammographically unsuspected multifocal or multicentric cancers in 28 patients (14%) and contralateral cancer in eight patients (4%) on ultrasound in a group of 194 invasive and in situ carcinomas. Selinko and colleagues,[27] in their study of 62 biopsy-proven cases of ILC, identified multicentricity or multifocality on ultrasound in 21% (13 of 62) of the patients.

The most common ultrasound appearances of ILC are predominantly hypoechoic masses with heterogeneous internal echoes, ill-defined, spiculated, or angular margins, and posterior acoustic shadowing (**Fig. 7**).[25–28] Current high-frequency transducers are able to demonstrate malignant features such as spiculations and microlobulations, which were not easily seen with the older 7.5-MHz transducers. Harmonic imaging may help to detect subtle hypoechoic masses and to accentuate posterior acoustic shadowing.

Selinko and colleagues[27] described the appearances of 62 cases of pure ILC. The most common sonographic appearance was a hypoechoic mass, associated with posterior acoustic shadowing (**Fig. 8**) in 36 cases (58%), and without posterior acoustic shadowing in 17 cases (27%). Posterior acoustic shadowing, without an associated mass, was seen in 7 cases (11%). A relatively well-defined mass was seen in 1 case (2%), and 1 lesion (2%) was sonographically occult. A characteristic infiltrative pattern appearing as an ill-defined area of altered, hypoechoic, heterogeneous echotexture with poorly defined margins was noted in 8 cases (13%). This pattern is thought to reflect the histologic pattern of the classic and the pleomorphic subtypes, with linear tumor cords that extend into the breast parenchyma in an infiltrative fashion. This infiltrative growth pattern is more readily identified on panoramic ultrasound views, with the heterogeneous echotexture of the abnormal tissue demonstrated in a background of normal breast tissue.

Waterman and colleagues demonstrated that histologic differentiation significantly influenced the ultrasound appearances of breast cancer. Waterman and colleagues described the ultrasound

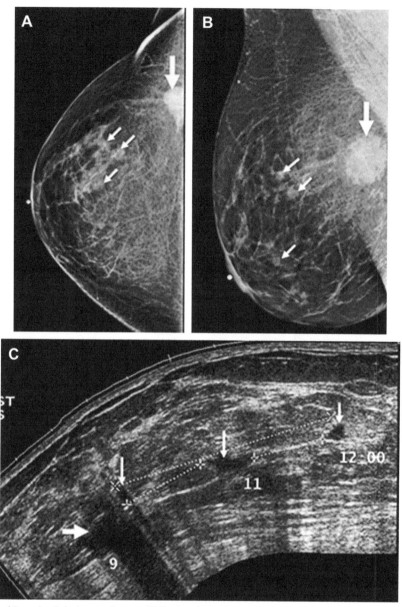

Fig. 6. Multifocal invasive lobular carcinoma (ILC). Craniocaudal (*A*) and mediolateral oblique (*B*) mammograms demonstrate a dominant mass (*large arrow*) and smaller masses (*small arrows*). (*C*) Panoramic ultrasound of the upper outer quadrant of the right breast demonstrates the dominant lesion (9 o'clock, *thick arrow*) and 3 smaller masses (at 10 o'clock, 11 o'clock, and 12 o'clock; *thin arrows*). The cursors indicate the distances between the lesions. The large mass and the smaller masses were proven to represent ILC on pathology.

morphology of 406 invasive breast cancers. The breast cancers were stratified into two groups: ILC (n = 69) and invasive tumors of other histologic differentiation (TOD) (n = 337). Waterman and colleagues described 10 sonographic criteria: shape, orientation, echogenicity, echo pattern, calcifications, margin, margin contour, lesion boundary, surrounding tissue, and posterior acoustic features. These features were compared in both groups. Waterman and colleagues[31] also analyzed the correlation between the measured sizes of the tumors on sonography and on pathology. On ultrasound, an irregular shape was found in 88% of ILCs, compared with 67% of TOD. Margins were indistinct in 94% of ILCs, compared with 76% of TOD. Posterior shadowing was observed in 84% of ILCs and 58% of TOD. Irregular margins, hyperechoic or isoechoic patterns, and architectural distortions were more frequent in ILCs than in TOD. Underestimation of

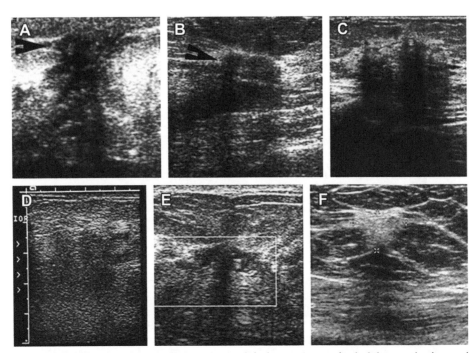

Fig. 7. Spectrum of ultrasound appearances in invasive lobular carcinoma (ILC). (*A*) Irregular hypoechoic mass (*arrowhead*) with spiculated margins and posterior acoustic shadowing. (*B*) Hypoechoic oval mass (*arrowhead*) with well-defined margins. (*C*) Hypoechoic masss with extensive posterior acoustic shadowing. (*D*) Ill-defined, subtle region of architectural distortion. (*Courtesy of* Dr Phan Huynh.) (*E*) Hypoechoic, wider-than-tall mass (outlined by box). (*F*) Hyperechoic mass (calipers). (*From* Whitman GJ, Huynh PT, Patel P, et al. Sonography of invasive lobular carcinoma. Ultrasound Clin 2007;1:654; with permission.)

tumor size by ultrasound was significantly more frequent in ILC than in TOD.

The ultrasound appearances of the various subtypes of ILC overlap considerably; however, certain subtypes are more likely to have a particular appearance on ultrasound. Classic ILC is most commonly seen on ultrasound as an area of focal shadowing without a discrete mass.Pleomorphic ILC is more typically seen as a shadowing mass. Signet ring, alveolar, and solid subtypes of ILC are more likely to be identified as lobulated or well-circumscribed masses.[14]

Cawson and colleagues, in their study of 62 screen-detected cases of ILC, described certain atypical appearances that may be seen in ILC. Cawson and colleagues found that a large proportion of ILCs had a wider-than-tall shape on ultrasound. A taller-than-wide shape, typically seen in malignant lesions, was seen in only 9 out of 37 ILCs (24%). Cawson and colleagues[32] found that ILC cases were less likely to be taller than wide when compared with IDC cases. The authors suggested that the flatter shape reflected the morphology of ILC, with the tumor cells spreading in a horizontal fashion along normal tissue planes, unlike IDC, which tends to grow across tissue planes.

Cawson and colleagues also described hyperechoic lesions as atypical findings in ILC. Cawson and colleagues[32] found that 21 of 37 (57%) ILCs were echogenic and showed that ILCs were nearly 10 times more likely to be hyperechoic when compared with IDCs. ILC infiltration into the surrounding tissues is suspected to cause an increase in reflective surfaces sonographically, resulting in increased internal echoes, and, thus, increasing the overall echogenicity of ILC.

THE ROLE OF SONOGRAPHY IN THE DIAGNOSIS OF AXILLARY LYMPH NODE METASATSES IN ILC

The prognosis and treatment of patients with invasive breast cancer is dependent on the axillary lymph node status. Ultrasound plays a vital role in the preoperative diagnosis of axillary lymph node metastases by identifying lymph nodes that have suspicious morphologic features. Cytologic confirmation of nodal metastases is then made by ultrasound-guided fine needle aspiration (FNA) in practices with good cytology support. If cytology support is not adequate, the axillary lymph nodes can be sampled by ultrasound-guided core biopsy.

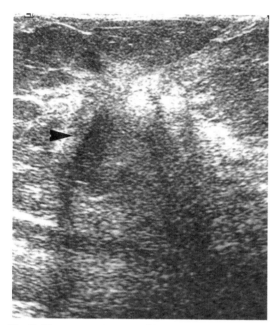

Fig. 8. Transverse ultrasound in a 40-year-old woman reveals an irregular hypoechoic mass (*arrowhead*) with associated posterior shadowing in the 11 o'clock position. Ultrasound-guided core needle biopsy demonstrated invasive lobular carcinoma (ILC).

If axillary lymph node metastases are confirmed, the patient can then proceed directly to axillary lymph node dissection instead of sentinel lymph node biopsy.[33]

Research has been performed to identify the predictors of axillary lymph node metastases on gray-scale ultrasound, contrast-enhanced ultrasound, and Doppler ultrasound. Many of these studies, however, consist of a heterogeneous group of various histologic types of primary breast cancers. One of the few studies consisting of pure ILC cases is a study by Boughey and colleagues.[34] Boughey and colleagues evaluated the reliability of ultrasound with FNA of the axillary lymph nodes in 217 patients with ILC. Preoperative ultrasound was negative in 137 patients (63%) and suspicious or indeterminate in 80 patients (37%). Ultrasound-guided FNA was performed in 76 (95%) of the 80 patients with indeterminate or suspicious findings on sonography. Comparison was made with the final pathology results obtained after axillary lymph node dissection. Boughey and colleagues[34] found that axillary ultrasound had a sensitivity of 52% (58 of 111), a specificity of 79% (84 of 106), a positive predictive value (PPV) of 73%, and a negative predictive value (NPV) of 61% in the identification of nodal metastases. In the subgroup of patients with indeterminate or suspicious lymph nodes on ultrasound, FNA was found to have a sensitivity

of 78% (43 of 55 patients), a specificity of 81% (17 of 21 patients), a PPV of 91%, and an NPV of 59%. Overall, nodal metastases were detected preoperatively by ultrasound with FNA in 43 of the 111 lymph node-positive patients. Therefore, the overall sensitivity of sonography with FNA for preoperative nodal staging of ILC patients was 39% (43 of 111 patients), with a specificity of 96% (102 of 106 patients), a PPV of 91%, and an NPV of 60%.

MAGNETIC RESONANCE IMAGING APPEARANCES OF INVASIVE LOBULAR CARCINOMA

The reported sensitivity of magnetic resonance imaging (MRI) in detecting ILC ranges from 83% to 100%.[35] MRI is particularly useful as an adjunctive tool to standard imaging techniques when clinical suspicion remains high despite negative mammographic and ultrasound examinations. Several studies have shown that MRI has the potential to affect the surgical management of known ILC. Mann and colleagues[36] conducted a retrospective cohort study of a consecutive series of 267 patients with ILC who had undergone breast-conserving surgery. Mann and colleagues found that re-excision rates after initial breast-conserving surgery were significantly lower in patients in whom preoperative breast MRI had been performed (9%) than in those who had not undergone preoperative MRI (27%). Mann and colleagues[36] also found that patients who had preoperative MRI scans had a lower final mastectomy rate than those who had not undergone preoperative MRI.

The potential of MRI to affect management is related to the fact that MRI has been found to be superior to other imaging modalities in accurately determining the size of lesions, defining the extent of disease involvement, and in detecting multifocality, multicentricity, and bilaterality. Accurate preoperative assessment of tumor size and disease extent is vital in staging of ILC, as these measurements help to determine the extent of surgical resection, predict response to chemotherapy, and help to select cases suitable for new nonsurgical treatments such as radiofrequency ablation, cryoablation, and focused ultrasound therapy.[37]

Mann and colleagues performed a study of 67 ILC lesions, correlating the appearances of the lesions on mammography, MRI and pathology. Mann and colleagues[37] found that MRI measurements correlated better with pathologic size than mammographic measurements. Underestimation of lesion size occurred significantly more often on mammography, compared with MRI. Overestimation of lesion size, on the other hand, occurred with equal frequency on mammography and MRI.

In a meta-analysis consisting of several studies, Mann and colleagues[35] reported on 3 studies that specifically correlated unifocality and multifocality seen on MRI with findings on pathology. Of the 67 cases, 7% were overestimated and described as multifocal but found to be unifocal on pathology. Conversely, 3% of the cases were underestimated as unifocal at MRI but were multifocal according to pathology. Two of the studies in the meta-analysis by Mann and colleagues,[35] one by Rodenko and colleagues and the other by Schelfout and colleagues, showed that MRI was more accurate in distinguishing single-quadrant from multicentric involvement. Out of a total of 46 patients in both studies, 2 cases of single quadrant disease were erroneously classified as multicentric on MRI but were unifocal on pathology and were thus overestimated. No cases were underestimated on MRI. In comparison, mammography in 42 of these patients resulted in overestimation of disease extent in 1 patient and underestimation in 15 patients. Four lesions were occult on mammography.[35]

Detection of concurrent additional lesions in the affected breast and the identification of contralateral cancers only visible on MRI were also analyzed in the meta-analysis by Mann and colleagues.[35] Additional malignant findings in the ipsilateral breast were present in 32% of 146 cases in 5 studies. Contralateral cancers only visible on MRI were present in 7% of 206 cases in 8 studies. MRI led to a change in surgical management in 28.3% of the cases.

As with other modalities, the appearance of ILC on MRI is variable. Qayyum and colleagues[38] described 3 morphologic patterns of ILC on MRI in a study of 13 pathologically proven cases (Fig. 9). The first MRI pattern was a discrete solitary mass with irregular margins (n = 4). The second pattern consisted of multiple small enhancing lesions arranged in clusters. In some cases, the multiple small enhancing foci were connected by enhancing strands, which correlated with noncontiguous tumor foci with malignant cells streaming in a single-file fashion in the breast stroma on pathology (n = 6). In other cases, the enhancing clusters were connected by nonenhancing intervening tissue, which correlated with small tumor aggregates separated by normal tissue on pathology (n = 2). The third pattern on MRI was seen in 1 patient as enhancing septations without a discrete mass (n = 1). On pathology, this pattern correlated with the appearance of tumor cells streaming in the breast stroma.

Schelfout and colleagues[39] described 4 major and 2 minor morphologic patterns on MRI in their study of 26 pathologically proven cases of ILC. The most common pattern (43%) was an irregular, spiculated, inhomogeneous mass, considered a major pattern. The second major pattern (29%) was a dominant, irregular, spiculated, heterogeneous lesion surrounded by 1 or more small enhancing foci. Multiple small enhancing foci with interconnecting and enhancing strands and architectural distortion were the 2 other major patterns, both described in 11% of the cases. The 2 minor patterns were demonstrated in 1 case (3%) of a focal irregular area of inhomogeneous enhancement and 1 negative MRI examination (3%).

Despite its superior imaging qualities, the role of MRI in staging invasive breast cancers remains controversial. Due to its relatively low specificity, breast MRI may create further diagnostic dilemmas by demonstrating enhancing lesions of uncertain significance, leading to additional percutaneous biopsies and/or surgical procedures. However, many centers have adopted MRI in local staging of ILC, especially when breast conserving surgery is planned, due to the high incidence of multifocality, multicentricity, and bilaterality in ILC.

COMPARATIVE ANALYSIS OF MAMMOGRAPHY, ULTRASOUND, AND MRI IN THE DIAGNOSIS OF ILC

McGhan and colleagues analyzed the findings in 70 women with ILC who underwent clinical breast examination (CBE), mammography, ultrasound, and MRI preoperatively. They noted that the sensitivities for the detection of ILC were 99% for MRI, 92% for ultrasound, 79% for mammography, and 63% for CBE. McGhan and colleagues[40] reported that additional suspicious lesions identified incidentally during MRI resulted in biopsies being performed in 39% of the cases, and all these biopsies revealed benign findings on pathology.

McGhan and colleagues also analyzed concordance rates for lesions measured by mammography, sonography, and MRI with the size of the tumor on final pathology. In contrast to the results of the meta-analysis by Mann and colleagues, which found that MRI correlated better with pathologic size than mammography, McGhan and colleagues found that mammography correlated best with pathology of all 3 imaging modalities. MRI was found to overestimate tumor size by 0.5 to 5.2 cm in 18 tumors (31%). However, no patients had an unnecessary mastectomy performed because of overestimation. MRI underestimated tumor size by more than 0.5 cm in 8 tumors

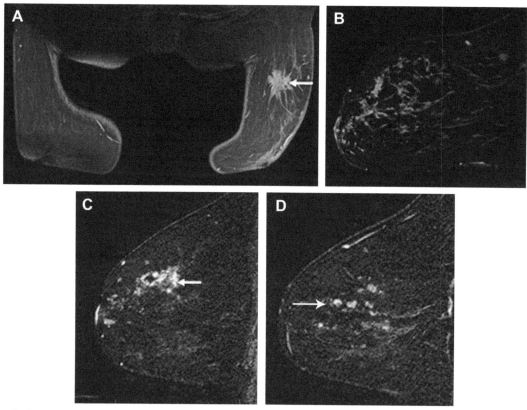

Fig. 9. Common appearances of invasive lobular carcinoma (ILC) on magnetic resonance imaging (MRI). (*A*) Bilateral axial dynamic contrast-enhanced MRI shows a solitary enhancing irregular mass (*arrow*) with spiculated margins. (*B*) Sagittal subtraction image demonstrates multiple small enhancing foci connected by enhancing septations. Sagittal subtraction images show a dominant enhancing mass (*C, short arrow*) and a cluster of several smaller masses (*D, long arrow*) that were shown to represent foci of ILC.

(14%); however, none of these patients required further surgery as a result of positive or close margins. McGhan and colleagues suggested that the lower rate of concordance between MRI and pathology may be related to the presence of surrounding LCIS which is known to cause enhancement. McGhan and colleagues[40] found surrounding LCIS at final pathology in 45% of tumors that were overestimated by MRI. Ultrasound was shown to have a tendency to underestimate tumor size.

Brem and colleagues[6] compared the sensitivity of mammography, sonography, MRI, and breast-specific gamma imaging (BSGI) using 99m-technetium sestamibi in the detection of ILC. They studied 26 women with biopsy-proven ILC who had undergone mammography and BSGI. Twenty-five patients had ultrasound examinations, and 12 patients underwent MRI. Final surgical pathology results were used as the gold standard. Brem and colleagues reported sensitivities of 79% for

mammography, 68% for sonography, and 83% for breast MRI. BSGI had a sensitivity of 93%. There was no statistically significant difference in the sensitivities of BSGI, MRI, sonography, or mammography, although there was a nonsignificant trend toward improved detection with BSGI.

SUMMARY

Ultrasound is a useful and affordable adjunctive tool in the diagnosis and local staging of ILC.[41] Compared to mammography, ultrasound is more sensitive for detecting ILC and better at demonstrating evidence of multifocal, multicentric, and bilateral disease. When used in conjunction with FNA, sonography helps to identify patients with axillary lymph node metastases preoperatively. Patients with proven axillary lymph node metastases then undergo axillary lymph node dissection rather than sentinel lymph node biopsy.

ACKNOWLEDGMENTS

The authors thank Barbara Almarez Mahinda and Joyce Bradley for assistance in manuscript preparation.

REFERENCES

1. Foote FW Jr, Stewart FW. A histologic classification of carcinoma of the breast. Surgery 1946;19:74–99.
2. Li CI, Daling JR. Changes in breast cancer incidence rates in the United States by histologic subtype and race/ethnicity, 1995 to 2004. Cancer Epidemiol Biomarkers Prev 2007;16:2773–80.
3. Krecke KN, Gisvold JJ. Invasive lobular carcinoma of the breast: mammographic findings and extent of disease at diagnosis in 184 patients. AJR Am J Roentgenol 1993;161:957–60.
4. Eheman CR, Shaw KM, Ryerson AB, et al. The changing incidence of in situ and invasive ductal and lobular breast carcinomas: United States, 1999–2004. Cancer Epidemiol Biomarkers Prev 2009;18:1763–9.
5. Kopans DB. Malignant lesions of the lobule. In: Kopans DB, editor. Breast imaging. Baltimore (MD): Lippincott Williams & Wilkins; 2007. p. 866–70.
6. Brem RF, Ioffe M, Rapelyea JA, et al. Invasive lobular carcinoma: detection with mammography, sonography, MRI, and breast-specific gamma imaging. AJR Am J Roentgenol 2009;192:379–83.
7. Li CI, Anderson BO, Daling JR, et al. Trends in incidence rates of invasive lobular and ductal breast carcinoma. JAMA 2003;289:1421–4.
8. Chen CL, Weiss NS, Newcomb P, et al. Hormone replacement therapy in relation to breast cancer. JAMA 2002;287:734–41.
9. Rosen PP. Invasive lobular carcinoma. In: Rosen PP, editor. Rosen's breast pathology. 2nd edition. Philadelphia: Lippincott, Williams & Wilkins; 2001. p. 627–38.
10. Ellis IO, Schnitt SJ, Sastre-Garau X, et al. Invasive breast carcinoma. In: Tavassoli FA, Devilee P, editors. World Health Organization classification of tumors. Pathology and genetic of tumors of the breast and female genital organs. Lyon (France): IARC Press; 2003. p. 23–6.
11. Orvieto E, Maiorano E, Bottiglieri L, et al. Clinico-pathologic characteristics of invasive lobular carcinoma of the breast: results of an analysis of 530 cases from a single institution. Cancer 2008;113: 1511–20.
12. Stavros AT. Malignant solid breast nodules. In: Stavros AT, editor. Breast ultrasound. Philadelphia: Lippincott Williams & Wilkins; 2004. p. 658.
13. Vargas AC, Lakhani SR, Simpson PT. Pleomorphic lobular carcinoma of the breast: molecular pathology and clinical impact. Future Oncol 2009;5:233–43.
14. Arpino G, Bardou VJ, Clark GM, et al. Infiltrating lobular carcinoma of the breast: tumor characteristics and clinical outcome. Breast Cancer Res 2004;6:R149–R56.
15. Winston CB, Hadar O, Teitcher JB, et al. Metastatic lobular carcinoma of the breast: patterns of spread in the chest, abdomen, and pelvis on CT. AJR Am J Roentgenol 2000;175:795–800.
16. Ferlicot S, Vincent-Salomon A, Médioni J, et al. Wide metastatic spreading in infiltrating lobular carcinoma of the breast. Eur J Cancer 2004;40:336–41.
17. Le Gal M, Ollivier L, Asselain B, et al. Mammographic features of 455 invasive lobular carcinomas. Radiology 1992;185:705–8.
18. Weinstein SP, Orel SG, Heller R, et al. MR imaging of the breast in patients with invasive lobular carcinoma. AJR Am J Roentgenol 2001;176:399–406.
19. Evans WP, Warren Burhenne LJ, Laurie L, et al. Invasive lobular carcinoma of the breast: mammographic characteristics and computer-aided detection. Radiology 2002;225:182–9.
20. The JS, Schilling KJ, Hoffmeister JW, et al. Detection of breast cancer with full-field digital mammography and computer-aided detection. AJR Am J Roentgenol 2009;192:337–40.
21. Hilleren DJ, Andersson IT, Lindholm K, et al. Invasive lobular carcinoma: mammographic findings in a 10-year experience. Radiology 1991;178:149–54.
22. Garnett S, Wallis M, Morgan G. Do screen-detected lobular and ductal carcinoma present with different mammographic features? Br J Radiol 2009;82:20–7.
23. Harvey JA, Fechner RE, Moore MM. Apparent ipsilateral decrease in breast size at mammography: a sign of infiltrating lobular carcinoma. Radiology 2000;214:883–9.
24. Jafri NF, Slanetz PJ. The shrinking breast: an unusual mammographic finding of invasive lobular carcinoma. Radiology Case Reports 2007;2:94.
25. Paramagul CP, Helvie MA, Adler DD. Invasive lobular carcinoma: sonographic appearance and role of sonography in improving diagnostic sensitivity. Radiology 1995;195:231–4.
26. Rissanen T, Tikkakoski T, Autio AL, et al. Ultrasonography of invasive lobular breast carcinoma. Acta Radiol 1998;39:285–91.
27. Selinko VL, Middleton LP, Dempsey PJ. Role of sonography in diagnosing and staging invasive lobular carcinoma. J Clin Ultrasound 2004;32: 323–32.
28. Butler RS, Venta LA, Wiley EL, et al. Sonographic evaluation of infiltrating lobular carcinoma. AJR Am J Roentgenol 1999;172:325–30.
29. Berg WA. Gilbreath PL. Multicentric and multifocal cancer: whole-breast US in preoperative evaluation. Radiology 2000;214:59–66.
30. Moon WK, Noh DY, Im JG. Multifocal, multicentric, and contralateral breast cancers: bilateral whole-breast

US in the preoperative evaluation of patients. Radiology 2002;224:569–76.

31. Watermann DO, Tempfer C, Hefler LA, et al. Ultrasound morphology of invasive lobular breast cancer is different compared with other types of breast cancer. Ultrasound Med Biol 2005;31:167–74.

32. Cawson JN, Law EM, Kavanagh AM. Invasive lobular carcinoma: sonographic features of cancers detected in a breast screen program. Australas Radiol 2001;45:25–30.

33. Mills P, Sever A, Weeks J, et al. Axillary ultrasound assessment in primary breast cancer: an audit of 653 cases. Breast J 2010;16:460–3.

34. Boughey JC, Middleton LP, Harker L, et al. Utility of ultrasound and fine-needle aspiration biopsy of the axilla in the assessment of invasive lobular carcinoma of the breast. Am J Surg 2007;194:450–5.

35. Mann RM, Hoogeveen YL, Blickman GB, et al. MRI compared to conventional diagnostic work-up in the detection and evaluation of invasive lobular carcinoma of the breast: a review of existing literature. Breast Cancer Res Treat 2008;107:1–14.

36. Mann RM, Loo CE, Wobbes T, et al. The impact of preoperative breast MRI on the re-excision rate in invasive lobular carcinoma of the breast. Breast Cancer Res Treat 2010;119:415–22.

37. Mann RM, Veltman J, Barentsz JO, et al. The value of MRI compared to mammography in the assessment of tumour extent in invasive lobular carcinoma of the breast. Eur J Surg Oncol 2008;34:135–42.

38. Qayyum A, Birdwell RL, Daniel BL, et al. MR imaging features of infiltrating lobular carcinoma of the breast: histopathologic correlation. AJR Am J Roentgenol 2002;178:1227–32.

39. Schelfout K, Van Goethem M, Kersschot E, et al. Preoperative breast MRI in patients with invasive lobular breast cancer. Eur Radiol 2004;14:1209–16.

40. McGhan LJ, Wasif N, Gray RJ, et al. Use of preoperative magnetic resonance imaging for invasive lobular cancer: good, better, but maybe not the best? Ann Surg Oncol 2010;17:255–62.

41. Whitman GJ, Huynh PT, Patel P, et al. Sonography of invasive lobular carcinoma. Ultrasound Clin 2007;1:645–60.

Ultrasound-Guided Breast Biopsy

Emily L. Sedgwick, MD

KEYWORDS

- Breast • Core needle biopsy • Ultrasound
- Fine-needle aspiration

At present, no imaging modality has been found to replace tissue sampling. For example, mammography has been reported to have a sensitivity ranging from 30% to 98%.[1] The specificity of mammography has been reported to be 93%.[2] The sensitivity of ultrasonography for the detection of breast cancer is usually reported in conjunction with mammography; where it has been reported independently, the sensitivity of ultrasonography is 83%, with a reported specificity of 34%.[1] Because of the imperfect sensitivity and specificity of current breast imaging modalities, radiologists are able to detect abnormalities but are not able to reliably exclude cancers. Biopsy is, therefore, often recommended. The positive predictive value of breast biopsies has been reported to be 12% in women younger than 40 years to as high as 46% for women in their late 70s.[3]

Before the advent of image-guided needle biopsies, women with breast imaging abnormalities underwent open surgical excision. The pooled sensitivity of open surgical biopsy has been estimated to be 98% to 99%.[4] In 1990, Parker and colleagues[5] published the first experience with stereotactic core needle biopsy. The first ultrasound-guided core needle biopsy was reported by Parker and colleagues[6] in 1993. Multiple studies have subsequently validated the fundamental role of image-guided breast biopsy in the care of women as an alternative to open surgical excision. Stereotactic core needle biopsy sensitivities have ranged from 97.8% to 99.2%.[4] Ultrasound-guided biopsy has been shown to have sensitivities that range from 92% to 100%.[7] Ultrasound-guided biopsy with an automated gun has a sensitivity of 97.7%, and use of a vacuum-assisted device with ultrasound guidance has a reported sensitivity of 96.5%.[4]

Benefits of image-guided biopsy over surgical excision include financial savings and decreased patient morbidity. Ultrasound-guided breast biopsy has been reported to be approximately 56% less expensive than open surgical biopsy, and stereotactic core needle biopsy has been shown to result in a cost saving of 39% compared with open surgical biopsy.[8] Regarding decreased morbidity, significant complications after image-guided core needle biopsy occur in fewer than 1% of patients.[4] Women who undergo image-guided biopsy do not need conscious sedation or general anesthesia and have improved cosmesis compared with women who have open surgical biopsy.[9] Image-guided biopsy has also been shown to decrease morbidity in women with breast cancer. Smith and colleagues[10] found that women with nonpalpable breast cancers underwent fewer surgical procedures if their initial diagnosis of cancer had been done via image-guided core needle biopsy rather than open surgical excision.

Ultrasonography is the technique preferred over stereotaxis for biopsy of masses because of its real-time assessment of needle placement, patient comfort, and greater accessibility to lesions. In addition, evaluation and sampling of suspicious axillary, internal mammary, and infraclavicular and supraclavicular lymph nodes can be performed if ultrasound guidance is used.[11] Ultrasound guidance does not use ionizing radiation. Occasionally, ultrasound guidance may be helpful for sampling calcifications in patients who cannot tolerate a stereotactic core needle biopsy. If ultrasound-guided biopsy of calcifications is performed, a specimen radiograph of the samples should be done to evaluate for the presence of the targeted calcifications.

Department of Radiology, Baylor College of Medicine, Baylor Plaza, MS 360, Houston, TX 77030, USA
E-mail address: sedgwick@bcm.edu

Ultrasound Clin 6 (2011) 327–333
doi:10.1016/j.cult.2011.05.001
1556-858X/11/$ – see front matter © 2011 Elsevier Inc. All rights reserved.

Once it has been decided that a patient should undergo ultrasound-guided core needle biopsy, patient positioning is performed. Careful consideration of patient positioning is essential because it affects the speed, accuracy, and safety of the procedure. Patients are placed supine but may be rolled into an oblique position to ensure that the needle path is parallel to the chest wall. Towels or a wedge may be placed under the patient's back, elbows, and knees for comfort and positioning. The biopsy table may be moved to assist in the optimal positioning of the patient and the physician, so that the ultrasound monitor is easily seen. The physician may stand on either side of the table, depending on the lesion location. A high-frequency transducer, preferably of 10 MHz or higher, is used. The physician may hold the transducer with one hand and the biopsy device with the other hand; alternatively, some physicians prefer that an assistant hold the ultrasound transducer. The lesion of interest is identified. An ink mark can be made on the skin along the edge of the transducer so the physician does not need to reidentify the lesion with each biopsy specimen. The needle path should be parallel to the chest wall to minimize the risk of pneumothorax and to visualize the entire length of the needle to ensure adequate sampling (**Fig. 1**).

The skin is sterilely prepped with povidone-iodine solution and anesthetized. In the author's clinic, 1% lidocaine is used as the local anesthetic for both the skin and along the biopsy needle path. Communication with the patient is key during the procedure for both patient comfort and compliance. A physician warns the patient when giving the local anesthetic and also allows the patient to hear the sound of the biopsy device, so that the patient does not move in surprise during tissue acquisition. If possible, the physician invites the patient to watch the procedure on the ultrasound monitor. Watching the procedure can distract patients during the biopsy, helping them to comply with the procedure.

If the lesion is close to the chest wall, a pool of lidocaine can be injected immediately dorsal to the target lesion to increase the distance between

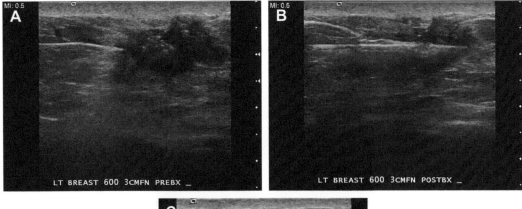

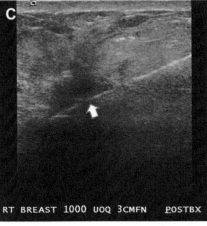

Fig. 1. (*A*) Correct needle placement. The biopsy needle is parallel to the chest wall and skin before the needle is deployed. (*B*) Correct needle placement. The biopsy needle passes through the mass, parallel to the chest wall and skin. (*C*) Bad needle placement. The angle of the biopsy needle is not parallel to the skin or chest wall. The site of skin entry should be more distal to the transducer. Biopsy yielded invasive ductal carcinoma. Arrow indicates needle.

the lesion and the chest wall. A nick is made in the skin with a scalpel, and the biopsy device is placed.

The choice of biopsy device is user dependent. Early work demonstrated high accuracy with 14-gauge automated biopsy devices.[6] More recent literature has confirmed the validity of 14-gauge automated biopsy devices compared with vacuum-assisted core needle biopsy devices.[12] If a 14-gauge automated biopsy device is used, at least 4 specimens should be obtained.[13]

The use of vacuum-assisted core needle biopsy has increased in many facilities. The vacuum-assisted devices require fewer samples, which may shorten the time of the biopsy. Another advantage of many vacuum-assisted biopsy devices is the single-insertion technique, obtaining multiple samples via a single insertion through the skin. The higher financial reimbursement for a vacuum-assisted core needle biopsy has also increased the use of this technique. An important drawback to the vacuum-assisted biopsy may be increased bleeding and hematoma formation, possibly because of the larger gauge of the needle.[4] Other studies, however, have disputed that there is a higher complication rate associated with vacuum-assisted core needle biopsy.[12]

Vacuum-assisted core needle biopsy has also been considered superior to 14-gauge automated core needle breast biopsy by some physicians because of lower underestimation rates. Underestimation is when a core needle biopsy identifies a histologic condition (eg, atypical ductal hyperplasia [ADH]) that is ultimately upstaged to a higher-grade lesion at surgical excision. Hoorntje and colleagues[14] found in their review of multiple studies that the high risk and ductal carcinoma in situ (DCIS) underestimation rates for 11-gauge vacuum-assisted core needle biopsy were 16% and 11%, respectively, as compared with 40% and 15%, respectively, for 14-gauge automated core needle biopsy. Bruening and colleagues,[4] in their review of multiple studies, found the underestimation of ADH by automated core needle biopsy to be 29.2% and underestimation of DCIS to be 35.5%. Underestimation rates for ultrasound-guided vacuum-assisted core needle biopsy could not be calculated in that review, but it was noted that underestimation rates of stereotactic vacuum-assisted core needle biopsy was lower than that of automated core needle biopsy.[4] Cho and colleagues[15] compared underestimation rates of ultrasound-guided 14-gauge automated core needle breast biopsy and 11-gauge vacuum-assisted core needle biopsy and found that vacuum-assisted core needle biopsy had lower ADH (20% vs 58%) and lower DCIS (41% vs 50%) underestimation rates.

More important than underestimation is miss rate, that is, the number of cancers missed by ultrasound-guided core needle biopsy. Some investigators have hypothesized that vacuum-assisted core needle biopsy misses fewer masses than 14-gauge automated core needle biopsy. This finding has not been proven. For ultrasound-guided 14-gauge automated core needle biopsy, the miss rate has been reported to range from 0% to 14%.[6,12] For ultrasound-guided vacuum-assisted core needle biopsy, a miss rate of 0.6% to 17% has been reported.[12,15,16]

In an effort to minimize missed cancers, attention to the ultrasound-guided biopsy technique is mandatory. As mentioned earlier, the needle path should be parallel to the chest wall to avoid pneumothorax; the needle should also be parallel to the transducer so it can be seen in its entirety. Parallel imaging of the needle often necessitates that the site of skin entry be at least 1 cm or more from the edge of the transducer. Deeper lesions may require a more-distant skin entry.[7] Once the core needle biopsy needle has been deployed, imaging of the needle along the needle path in the lesion and its orthogonal correlate in the lesion should be obtained to document satisfactory needle placement (**Fig. 2**).[7] Attention must be paid to adjacent relevant structures, such as large blood vessels or breast implants. Color Doppler can be used to evaluate the needle path and nearby structures that may cause unnecessary bleeding.

A mass close to the wall of a breast implant must be biopsied with caution. Implant rupture must be discussed in detail with the patient as part of the informed consent before the procedure. The blade of the scalpel could be turned 180° to keep the scalpel blade parallel to the implant wall when performing the dermotomy. The needle must be parallel to the implant wall at all times. It may be helpful to watch the needle tip with the ultrasound transducer at skin entry and slowly advance the biopsy needle to the edge of the target. If resistance is met, placement of an outer sheath may be helpful for better needle control. Alternatively, a gentle turning of the wrist while advancing the needle may be of use. If the implant is saline, rupture may be clinically apparent. Postprocedure mammograms can be obtained to document no change in implant contour when compared with preprocedure mammograms in an effort to demonstrate that the implant was not affected by the needle biopsy (**Fig. 3**).

Once the breast biopsy has been performed, ultrasound-guided sampling of axillary lymph nodes may be done if suspicious lymph nodes are identified. Because 97% of positive sentinel lymph nodes are found in the axilla, specific attention

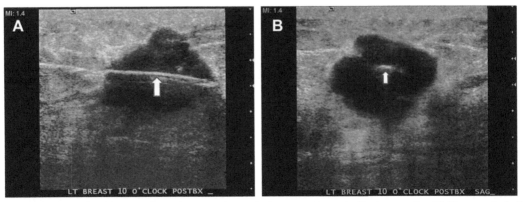

Fig. 2. (A) The length of the needle as it passes through the mass. Arrow indicates needle. (B) The needle in the mass from an orthogonal view. Biopsy yielded invasive ductal carcinoma. Arrow indicates needle.

should be paid to the axilla.[17] If an axillary lymph node can be demonstrated to be malignant by percutaneous sampling, the patient need not undergo the additional radiation exposure of sentinel lymph node biopsy and can proceed directly to axillary lymph node dissection, which decreases the duration for which the patient is ultimately under anesthesia and the duration for which the patient occupies the operating room (**Fig. 4**).

Two methods of ultrasound-guided core needle sampling are in current use: fine-needle aspiration (FNA) and core needle biopsy. FNA is not considered a reliable method for evaluation of breast masses by some investigators because it requires highly trained radiologists and cytologists who can correctly prepare and interpret the slides and then correlate the cytologic findings with the radiological findings.[18] FNA of lymph nodes has been demonstrated to have a sensitivity of 68% and specificity of 100%.[19] Others argue that FNA has an acceptable sensitivity and confers a cost benefit over conventional sentinel lymph node biopsy, but no studies, to date, have compared the costs of FNA with that of core needle biopsy of axillary lymph nodes.[20]

The sensitivity of 14-gauge ultrasound-guided core needle biopsy of suspicious axillary lymph nodes has been reported to be 94%, with a negative predictive value of 89%.[21] Complications from ultrasound-guided core needle biopsy of axillary lymph nodes are low.[21] Given the higher number of operators skilled in the procedure and higher

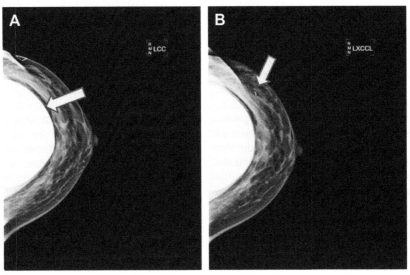

Fig. 3. (A) Preprocedure mammogram with implant. Arrow indicates implant margin. (B) Postprocedure mammogram with clip and unchanged implant contour. Arrow indicates clip.

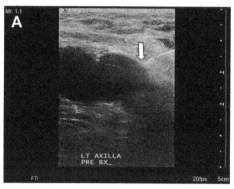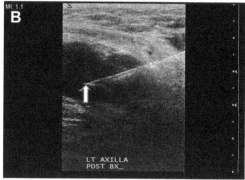

Fig. 4. (A) Axillary lymph node biopsy. A 14-gauge core needle biopsy needle tip is adjacent to the lymph node. Arrow indicates needle tip. (B) Axillary lymph node biopsy. A 14-gauge core needle biopsy needle tip is in the axillary lymph node. Biopsy yielded malignant cells. Arrow indicates needle tip.

sensitivity of ultrasound-guided core needle biopsy over FNA of breast masses, ultrasound-guided core needle biopsy of suspicious axillary lymph nodes is a reasonable method to sample lymph nodes, thereby obviating sentinel lymph node biopsy.

After tissue samples have been obtained, a marker may be placed. Tissue markers have been used with increasing frequency because of rising use of neoadjuvant therapy for breast cancer. Tissue markers often have characteristic shapes, and many may be imbedded in echogenic material for identification under ultrasound guidance and for hemostasis (**Fig. 5**). Different-shaped markers can be useful in patients with several lesions, and marker shape can be discussed in the radiology report. However, markers have been reported to migrate; so, a postprocedure mammogram is recommended to ensure that the marker accurately depicts the area of biopsy and to demonstrate that the sonographic target correlates with the mammographic area of concern.[22]

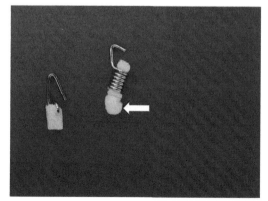

Fig. 5. Examples of markers. Markers may be associated with a polymer or collagen for improved visualization under ultrasound. Arrow indicates polymer.

Once the lesion has been biopsied and a marker placed, the tissue is sent for analysis. When the histologic results are reported, it is incumbent on the radiologist to evaluate the histologic results and decide whether the results are concordant with the imaging findings. If the results are concordant, follow-up is 1 of the 2 scenarios. If the malignant results are concordant with the imaging findings, clinical management of the malignancy is recommended. If the benign results are concordant with the benign imaging findings, a short-term follow-up ultrasonography is recommended in 6 months to ensure that no missed cancers are overlooked. The pooled negative likelihood ratio of ultrasound-guided biopsy was 0.030 to 0.036; hence, a 6-month follow-up ultrasonography is recommended.[4]

If the radiologist determines that the imaging findings are discordant with the histologic results, 2 scenarios are encountered. Imaging findings may have indicated a benign histologic condition, but malignant histologic results were found. In this case, further action should be performed based on the histologic results. If imaging findings were suspicious for malignancy, but the histologic results were benign, a repeat biopsy is recommended. In the author's institution, the repeat biopsy is performed via ultrasound-guided wire localization and surgical excision.

The final scenario involves high-risk lesions. If a high-risk lesion (eg, radial scar, atypia, mucocele) is described in the histology report, the radiologist and pathologist discuss the results and decide the management together. If there is uncertainty, the patient's case is presented to the multidisciplinary breast tumor board for treatment recommendations.

Once the radiology/histology concordance is determined, the results and follow-up recommendations are communicated to the patient and referring physician. Documentation of the communication with the patient and referring physician is recommended. This documentation can be performed as a note in the patient's medical record or as an addendum to the biopsy report.

As the practice of ultrasound-guided core needle biopsy has become more prevalent, physicians are extending its boundaries to include treatment. Although women with biopsy-proven fibroadenoma do not need surgical excision of the known fibroadenoma, many women dislike the palpable lump and request removal. Traditionally, this removal has required open surgical excision. Now that ultrasound-guided core needle biopsy has been shown to have a reliably high sensitivity and specificity for the detection of malignancy, many have used the large-core vacuum-assisted ultrasound-guided needle as a minimally invasive tool to remove the offending benign lesion with successful results.[23] Radiofrequency thermal ablation using ultrasound guidance has been described to treat both benign and malignant lesions with early successful results.[24,25] Ultrasound-guided balloons have been used to deliver local radiotherapy.[26]

Ultrasound-guided core needle biopsy was originally described in 1993. Since then, it has been shown to be a reliable, even preferred, alternative to open surgical biopsy. This technique should be the modality of choice for any breast or axillary sonographic abnormality requiring tissue sampling. The high sensitivity and reproducibility of this technique make ultrasound-guided core needle biopsy a low-cost procedure that minimizes patient morbidity. Attention to the technique, radiology/histology concordance, and follow-up are necessary to minimize any false-negative biopsy results. As ultrasound-guided core needle biopsy gains wider acceptance, its therapeutic uses (such as removal of masses) are becoming more prevalent.

REFERENCES

1. Berg WA, Gutierrez L, NessAiver MS, et al. Diagnostic accuracy of mammography, clinical examination, US, and MR imaging in preoperative assessment of breast cancer. Radiology 2004;233(3):830–49.

2. Burhenne HJ, Burhenne LW, Goldberg F, et al. Interval breast cancers in the Screening Mammography Program of British Columbia: analysis and classification. AJR Am J Roentgenol 1994;162(5):1067–71 [discussion: 1072–5].

3. Kopans DB, Moore RH, McCarthy KA, et al. Positive predictive value of breast biopsy performed as a result of mammography: there is no abrupt change at age 50 years. Radiology 1996;200(2):357–60.

4. Bruening W, Fontanarosa J, Tipton K, et al. Systematic review: comparative effectiveness of core-needle and open surgical biopsy to diagnose breast lesions. Ann Intern Med 2010;152(4):238–46.

5. Parker SH, Lovin JD, Jobe WE, et al. Stereotactic breast biopsy with a biopsy gun. Radiology 1990; 176(3):741–7.

6. Parker SH, Jobe WE, Dennis MA, et al. US-guided automated large-core breast biopsy. Radiology 1993;187(2):507–11.

7. Youk JH, Kim EK, Kim MJ, et al. Missed breast cancers at US-guided core needle biopsy: how to reduce them. Radiographics 2007;27(1):79–94.

8. Liberman L, Feng TL, Dershaw DD, et al. US-guided core breast biopsy: use and cost-effectiveness. Radiology 1998;208(3):717–23.

9. Ramachandran N. Breast intervention: current and future roles. Imaging 2008;20(3):176–84.

10. Smith DN, Christian R, Meyer JE. Large-core needle biopsy of nonpalpable breast cancers. The impact on subsequent surgical excisions. Arch Surg 1997; 132(3):256–9 [discussion: 260].

11. Whitman GJ, Erguvan-Dogan B, Yang WT, et al. Ultrasound-guided breast biopsies. Ultrasound Clin 2006;1: 603–15.

12. Philpotts LE, Hooley RJ, Lee CH. Comparison of automated versus vacuum-assisted biopsy methods for sonographically guided core biopsy of the breast. AJR Am J Roentgenol 2003;180(2):347–51.

13. Fishman JE, Milikowski C, Ramsinghani R, et al. US-guided core-needle biopsy of the breast: how many specimens are necessary? Radiology 2003;226(3): 779–82.

14. Hoorntje LE, Peeters PH, Mali WP, et al. Vacuum-assisted breast biopsy: a critical review. Eur J Cancer 2003;39(12):1676–83.

15. Cho N, Moon WK, Cha JH, et al. Sonographically guided core biopsy of the breast: comparison of 14-gauge automated gun and 11-gauge directional vacuum-assisted biopsy methods. Korean J Radiol 2005;6(2):102–9.

16. Cassano E, Urban LA, Pizzamiglio M, et al. Ultrasound-guided vacuum-assisted core breast biopsy: experience with 406 cases. Breast Cancer Res Treat 2007;102(1):103–10.

17. Krag D, Weaver D, Ashikaga T, et al. The sentinel node in breast cancer—a multicenter validation study. N Engl J Med 1998;339(14):941–6.

18. Abe H, Schmidt RA, Sennett CA, et al. US-guided core needle biopsy of axillary lymph nodes in patients with breast cancer: why and how to do it. Radiographics 2007;27(Suppl 1):S91–9.

19. Altomare V, Guerriero G, Carino R, et al. Axillary lymph node echo-guided fine-needle aspiration cytology enables breast cancer patients to avoid

a sentinel lymph node biopsy. Preliminary experience and a review of the literature. Surg Today 2007;37(9):735–9.

20. Genta F, Zanon E, Camanni M, et al. Cost/accuracy ratio analysis in breast cancer patients undergoing ultrasound-guided fine-needle aspiration cytology, sentinel node biopsy, and frozen section of node. World J Surg 2007;31(6):1155–63.

21. Abe H, Schmidt RA, Kulkarni K, et al. Axillary lymph nodes suspicious for breast cancer metastasis: sampling with US-guided 14-gauge core-needle biopsy—clinical experience in 100 patients. Radiology 2009;250(1):41–9.

22. Esserman LE, Cura MA, DaCosta D. Recognizing pitfalls in early and late migration of clip markers after imaging-guided directional vacuum-assisted biopsy. Radiographics 2004;24(1):147–56.

23. Sperber F, Blank A, Metser U, et al. Diagnosis and treatment of breast fibroadenomas by ultrasound-guided vacuum-assisted biopsy. Arch Surg 2003; 138(7):796–800.

24. Kaufman CS, Littrup PJ, Freeman-Gibb LA, et al. Office-based cryoablation of breast fibroadenomas with long-term follow-up. Breast J 2005;11(5):344–50.

25. Hayashi AH, Silver SF, van der Westhuizen NG, et al. Treatment of invasive breast carcinoma with ultrasound-guided radiofrequency ablation. Am J Surg 2003;185(5):429–35.

26. Vicini F, Beitsch PD, Quiet CA, et al. Three-year analysis of treatment efficacy, cosmesis, and toxicity by the American Society of Breast Surgeons MammoSite Breast Brachytherapy Registry Trial in patients treated with accelerated partial breast irradiation (APBI). Cancer 2008;112(4):758–66.

Ultrasonography and Ultrasound-Guided Biopsy of Breast Calcifications

Phan T. Huynh, MD

KEYWORDS

- Ultrasonography • Ultrasound-guided biopsy
- Breast calcifications • BI-RADS 4/5

Breast calcifications are frequently identified on mammography in the screening and diagnostic settings. The vast majority of these calcifications can be characterized as benign based on their mammographic appearances. Typically benign calcifications include skin, vascular, secretory, coarse, dystrophic, eggshell, lucent-centered, milk of calcium, round, and punctuate calcifications.[1] However, calcifications may also indicate the presence of ductal carcinoma in situ (DCIS) and/or invasive breast cancer. Calcifications are classified as suspicious or highly suggestive of malignancy based on morphology, distribution, interval change, and associated findings, such as a masses or architectural distortions. Calcifications are the dominant feature in 90% of DCIS cases,[2] and the incidence of DCIS has increased considerably (by 9% per year) from 1999 to 2004, due to mammographic screening.[3]

Quality mammography is essential for the detection of breast calcifications. Full-field digital mammography provides improved contrast resolution compared with film-screen mammography. When indeterminate calcifications are detected on screening mammograms, magnification views, including true lateral projections, should be obtained. If the indeterminate calcifications are classified as suspicious (Breast Imaging Reporting and Data System [BI-RADS] category 4) or highly suggestive (BI-RADS category 5) of malignancy, histopathological confirmation can be usually accomplished with stereotactic biopsy. This article discusses the increased use of ultrasonography in the evaluation and management of BI-RADS 4 and 5 breast calcifications.[1]

EVALUATION OF BREAST CALCIFICATIONS ON MAMMOGRAPHY

Liberman and colleagues[4] prospectively evaluated 492 nonpalpable mammographically detected lesions with BI-RADS (second edition) descriptors and assessment categories. Among the morphologic descriptors for breast calcifications, Liberman and colleagues[4] found the following frequencies of carcinoma: 9% for punctate calcifications, 26% for amorphous calcifications, 41% for pleomorphic calcifications, and 81% for linear calcifications. Distribution descriptors were associated with the following frequencies of carcinoma: 0% for diffuse, 36% for clustered, 46% for regional, 68% for linear, and 74% for segmental distributions.

Burnside and colleagues[5] performed a retrospective study of 115 consecutive women who underwent image-guided biopsy of breast calcifications using the descriptors in BI-RADS (fourth edition). Coarse heterogeneous (irregular, conspicuous calcifications that are generally larger than 0.5 mm) were associated with a 7% probability of malignancy. Amorphous calcifications were associated with a 13% probability of malignancy. Fine pleomorphic (varying in sizes and shapes, usually <0.5 mm in diameter) calcifications had a 29% probability of malignancy, and fine linear

Department of Radiology, St Luke's Episcopal Hospital, MC 2-270, 6720 Bertner Avenue, Houston, TX 77030, USA
E-mail address: phuynh1@sleh.com

Ultrasound Clin 6 (2011) 335–343
doi:10.1016/j.cult.2011.03.011
1556-858X/11/$ – see front matter © 2011 Elsevier Inc. All rights reserved.

calcifications were associated with the highest risk (53%) for malignancy. The distribution descriptors were found to be highly predictive of malignancy, with increasing risks from diffuse, scattered, to clustered, to linear and segmental distributions. Calcifications with known interval change were associated with a statistically significant increased risk of malignancy (32%) as compared with calcifications for which stability was unknown (13%).[5]

Calcifications assigned to BI-RADS category 4 were associated with 33% probability of malignancy, whereas BI-RADS 5 calcifications had a 78% probability of malignancy. Furthermore, invasive breast cancers were significantly more likely to be found with BI-RADS 5 calcifications (24%) than with BI-RADS 4 calcifications (8%).[5]

Calcifications account for approximately 50% of the biopsies of nonpalpable breast lesions.[3] Stereotactic vacuum-assisted biopsy is the accepted standard of care for biopsy of breast calcifications that are suspicious or highly suggestive of malignancy. Of the biopsied calcifications, 35% to 70% of malignancies represent DCIS. If DCIS is diagnosed with imaging-guided percutaneous biopsy and invasive cancer is found at surgical excision, the term underestimation is applied. The underestimation rate (defined as the rate of high risks lesions diagnosed at core biopsy and upgraded to DCIS or invasive cancer at surgery coupled with the rate of DCIS diagnosed at core biopsy upgraded to invasive cancer at surgery) for DCIS found at stereotactic automated large-core 14-gauge needle biopsy is 15% to 36%.[6] The use of 11-gauge vacuum-assisted biopsy devices lowered the histologic underestimation rate of DCIS to 5%.[7] However, the underestimation rate of DCIS for calcifications highly suggestive of malignancy was 26.7%, even with the use of 11-gauge vacuum-assisted biopsy devices.[8] More recently, a retrospective study by Eby and colleagues[9] showed the underestimation rate of DCIS to be 21.6% with the use of 9-gauge vacuum-assisted biopsy devices.

USE OF ULTRASONOGRAPHY IN THE EVALUATION OF BREAST CALCIFICATIONS

Ultrasonography has traditionally been used in characterizing breast masses. Ultrasonography can also be used to provide imaging guidance for interventional procedures targeting suspicious, sonographically visible calcifications. Advances in state-of-the-art, high-frequency transducers have led to improved contrast and resolution. Yang and colleagues[10] retrospectively studied 84 consecutive patients with 89 histologically proven breast cancers with mammography and ultrasonography.

Yang and colleagues used a 10- to 5-MHz broadband transducer to evaluate the ability of ultrasonography to detect calcifications within breast cancers. Ultrasonography was found to be highly sensitive (95%) in detecting calcifications in cancerous masses, likely due to the hypoechoic background that allowed for enhanced visualization of the bright echogenic calcifications.

Moon and colleagues[11] prospectively evaluated 94 consecutive patients with 100 mammographically detected clusters of calcifications with ultrasonography prior to surgical breast biopsy. There were 62 benign lesions and 38 malignancies (30 DCIS and 8 invasive cancers). Malignant breast masses associated with calcifications were more likely to be detected by ultrasonography than benign breast masses. Regarding malignant clusters of calcifications larger than 10 mm, ultrasonography showed associated breast masses in all 25 cases. Breast masses associated with calcifications were more frequently seen with invasive breast cancer rather than with DCIS. The typical findings associated with invasive breast cancers on sonography included irregular or lobular shapes, hypoechogenicity, microlobulated or ill-defined margins, and heterogeneous echotexture. Among the subtypes of DCIS, the comedo variant, typically associated with higher grade cancers, was more frequently associated with sonographically visible breast masses (**Fig. 1**) compared with other subtypes. The ultrasound findings of DCIS were nonspecific. Nonetheless, it was worth noting that breast masses associated with DCIS were more likely to be wider than tall, mildly hypoechoic, and associated with normal acoustic transmission—features usually associated with benignity on ultrasonography.

Hashimoto reported 5 general appearances of DCIS on sonography: calcifications (**Figs. 2** and **3**), solid masses, solid masses associated with fluid collections, dilated ducts (**Fig. 4**) and clusters of cysts. Finding DCIS in a cluster of small cysts is extremely uncommon, and the microcysts associated with DCIS tend to be irregular in size and shape.[12]

Soo and colleagues prospectively evaluated 105 patients with 111 suspicious clusters of calcifications without other mammographic abnormalities with targeted ultrasonography before biopsy. Twenty-six lesions (23%) were seen as masses or ducts with calcifications and subsequently biopsied under sonographic guidance with either a multipass automated gun and a 14-gauge needle or a handheld 11-gauge vacuum-assisted biopsy device. Eighty-five lesions (77%) were not identified sonographically and were subsequently biopsied under stereotactic guidance. The diameters

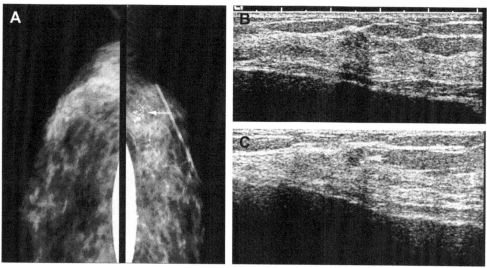

Fig. 1. (*A*) Bilateral implant displaced craniocaudal views demonstrate segmental, heterogeneous calcifications in the lateral left breast (*arrow*). (*B*, *C*) Ultrasonogram shows two separate, ill-defined, hypoechoic masses (*cursors* in *B* and *arrow* in *C*) in the middle and the posterior upper outer left breast associated with the heterogeneous calcifications seen on mammography. Ultrasound-guided biopsy confirmed the diagnosis of extensive high-grade DCIS with invasive foci in this patient with silicone breast implants.

of the clusters of calcifications identified on ultrasonography were significantly larger when compared with the calcification clusters not seen on ultrasonograms. Also, the calcification clusters seen on sonography were composed of more calcifications when compared with the calcification groups not seen on ultrasonography. The sonographically identified lesions were more likely to be malignant when compared with those not seen on sonography. Calcifications depicted on sonography were shown as echogenic foci within hypoechoic or isoechoic masses or within hypoechoic dilated ducts. The masses were irregular or lobular, and were likely wider than tall. Of interest, 72% of the wider than tall masses in this group of lesions were malignant. Of all the malignant lesions, those identified on sonography were more likely to be invasive than those not seen on sonography. There was less underestimation of the extent of disease in the sonographically identified and biopsied calcifications than with the lesions not seen on ultrasonography.[13]

ULTRASOUND TECHNIQUE FOR VISUALIZATION OF BREAST CALCIFICATIONS

Accurate correlation of mammographic and sonographic findings, and attention to detail to maximize sonographic resolution and contrast, are the keys to visualization of breast calcifications. As calcifications are usually detected first on mammography, one needs to be able to identify the mammographic findings in 3 dimensions within

the breast, as there are known variations in patient positioning with different modalities. The patient is usually standing or sitting for mammography, positioned supine or supine oblique for ultrasonography, and positioned prone for magnetic resonance imaging (MRI). The mammogram usually comprises medial-lateral oblique (MLO) and craniocaudal (CC) views. The concept of triangulation is used to assess where a potential abnormality moves from the MLO (at various angles parallel to the patient's pectoral muscle) view to the true lateral (90°) position. Lateral lesions move lower from the CC view to the MLO view to the true lateral view. The location of a lesion can be described in terms of quadrant, clock face, depth, or relationships to fixed landmarks such as the nipple or the chest wall. Targeted ultrasonography of a mammographic finding should also assess the surrounding background environment. For example, a lesion located in the retroglandular fat region on mammography should not be seen as a lesion surrounded by fibroglandular tissue on sonography. High-frequency (>10 MHz) transducers should be used. To maximize resolution, the focal zone needs to be adjusted to the region of interest. Spatial compounding may be useful and may improve contrast resolution.

ULTRASOUND-GUIDED BIOPSY OF BREAST CALCIFICATIONS

Advantages of ultrasound-guided biopsies over stereotactic breast biopsies and surgical procedures

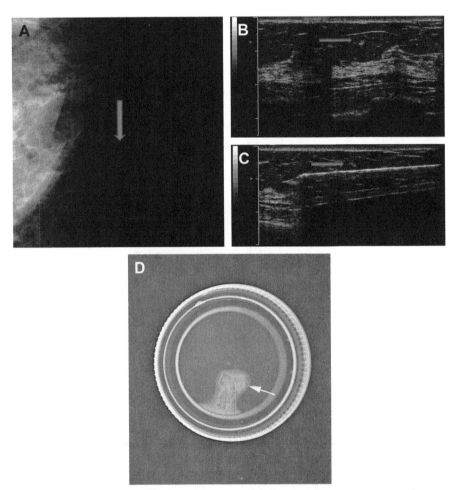

Fig. 2. (*A*) Magnification craniocaudal view demonstrates a small cluster of amorphous calcifications (*arrow*) in the subareolar medial left breast in a 48-year-old woman who was not a candidate for stereotactic biopsy, due to her inability to lay prone. (*B*) Targeted ultrasonogram shows a subtle cluster of echogenic foci (*arrow*). (*C*) The vacuum-assisted biopsy device is placed just below the targeted calcifications (*arrow*). (*D*) Specimen radiography confirms the presence of calcifications (*arrow*), shown to represent benign fibrocystic changes on pathology.

include lack of ionizing radiation, wider availability of ultrasound machines, and increased patient comfort. Ultrasound-guided procedures can also be performed quickly and are less costly than stereotactic procedures. Before undertaking ultrasound-guided procedures, all available imaging (ultrasonography, mammography, and MRI) studies should be reviewed. The targeted, sonographically visible lesions are then classified according to BI-RADS categories. Lesions designated as BI-RADS 3 (probably benign, having a <2% probability of malignancy) are appropriately managed with short-term imaging surveillance (usually at 6-month intervals for at least 2 years). Selected BI-RADS 3 lesions may be managed with imaging-guided percutaneous biopsy if a patient is unable to return for short-term imaging surveillance. Additional reasons for performing a percutaneous biopsy on BI-RADS 3 lesions include patient anxiety, pregnancy, and referring physicians' preferences.[1]

Preprocedural assessments and preparations are essential in maximizing the success of ultrasound-guided breast biopsies. All prior imaging studies (including mammography, breast ultrasonography, breast MRI, γ-specific breast imaging, computed tomography [CT], and positron emission tomography [PET]) should be reviewed. The radiologist who performs imaging-guided procedures should have finalized a BI-RADS assessment, independent of the original BI-RADS classification given by the interpreting radiologist. The use of subcategories 4a, 4b, and 4c is encouraged. At St Luke's Episcopal Hospital, the probabilities of malignancy are estimated to be

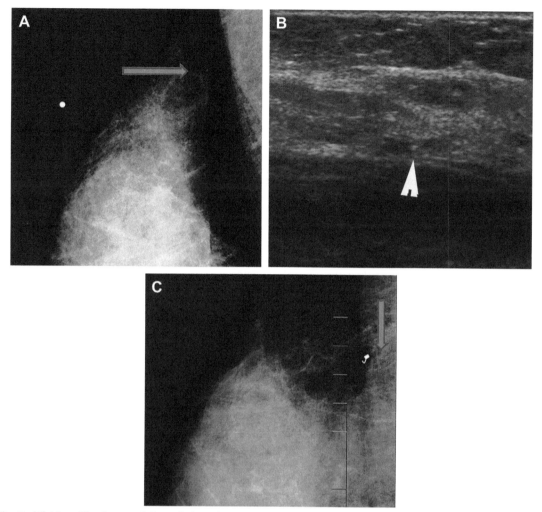

Fig. 3. (*A*) Magnification mediolateral view shows a cluster of heterogeneous calcifications (*arrow*) in the right axillary tail in a 42-year-old woman with a reported palpable abnormality (radiopaque marker) in the upper outer right breast. (*B*) Ultrasonogram of the region of the reported palpable abnormality did not show a sonographic correlate. The suspicious calcifications seen mammographically are visualized as a cluster of echogenic foci (*arrowhead*). (*C*) Ultrasound-guided biopsy of the echogenic foci was performed with a 14-gauge cutting needle, confirming the diagnosis of high-grade DCIS. Postbiopsy mammogram demonstrates appropriate clip placement, in the region of the targeted calcifications (*arrow*).

10% for 4a lesions, 25% for 4b lesions, and 50% for 4c lesions. When lesions are categorized appropriately as 4c, they need to be sampled adequately to minimize false negatives. Vacuum-assisted biopsy devices should be used if available, and a large number of specimens should be obtained. Suspicious or highly suspicious breast calcifications are usually biopsied under stereotactic guidance. Ultrasound-guided biopsy should be considered for patients with highly suspicious calcification groups measuring greater than 3 cm, associated with a background of heterogeneously dense fibroglandular tissue. If a suspicious sonographically visible mass is found, the chance of invasive disease increases and the underestimation rate decreases. On occasion, stereotactic biopsy of suspicious calcifications may be difficult in patients with thin breasts (thickness <3 cm), breast implants, or with lesions located in the subareolar (see **Fig. 2**) or the posterior (see **Fig. 3**) regions. Patients may weigh greater than the limit of the prone stereotactic biopsy table, precluding the performance of stereotactic biopsy procedures. These difficult cases are often referred for needle localization and surgical excisional biopsies. At St Luke's Episcopal Hospital a careful, directed ultrasound examination may be performed for the possibility

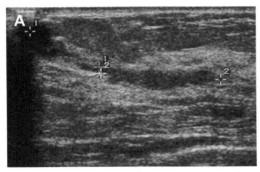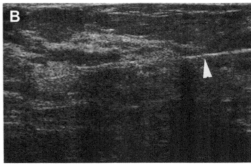

Fig. 4. (*A*) Ultrasonogram of a 50-year-old woman with bloody nipple discharge shows an abnormal, irregularly dilated duct (*cursors*). (*B*) Vacuum-assisted biopsy (biopsy device noted by *arrowhead*) under sonographic guidance was used to sample the duct, confirming the diagnosis of DCIS.

of visualizing and biopsying calcifications under sonographic guidance.

A patient questionnaire regarding the use of anticoagulants, aspirin, and/or nonsteroidal anti-inflammatory drugs is obtained at the time of scheduling for the invasive procedures. Whenever possible, patients are advised to refrain from anticoagulants for a week before the day of the invasive procedures. The risks, benefits, and alternatives to ultrasound-guided breast biopsy are then discussed with the patient before obtaining informed consent. Patients are placed in the supine position for medial lesions and in the supine oblique position for lateral lesions. A pillow or a triangular foam wedge can be placed under the patient's shoulder to provide support for the patient in the supine oblique position. The physician operator is usually positioned at the level of the patient's abdomen. On occasion, it may be advantageous for the operator to be positioned at the level of the patient's head (**Fig. 5**). For example, a right-handed operator positioned at the level of the head of the patient may approach medial left breast lesions medially to laterally, maneuvering the needle parallel to the patient's chest wall.

The operator should always be situated comfortably for the duration of the ultrasound-guided biopsy procedure. The skin in the region of interest is cleansed with povidone-iodine solution. The transducer is soaked in 70% isopropyl alcohol for several minutes before and after the procedure. The isopropyl alcohol serves as a disinfectant and as an acoustic coupling agent, eliminating the need for sterile gel. Local anesthesia with lidocaine buffered with sodium bicarbonate (at a 1 to 10 ratio) is administered subcutaneously and along the projected path of the biopsy needle. For ultrasound-guided vacuum-assisted biopsies, lidocaine can be administered via an 18-gauge hypodermic needle below and past the targeted

lesion. This maneuver creates easier paths for the larger 8- to 9-gauge vacuum-assisted biopsy devices, especially in patients with dense fibro-glandular tissue. Ultrasound-guided core biopsies can be performed with automated spring-loaded cutting needles, vacuum-assisted biopsy devices, and "hybrid" biopsy devices (vacuum-assisted devices without cables, requiring reinsertion for additional sampling). Automated long throw (2.2 cm) 14 gauge cutting needles are used most commonly, and in general, an average of 5 cores is obtained. A disadvantage of the use of automated cutting needles is the removal of the needle from the breast after each core to retrieve the specimen and the subsequent reinsertion of the needle for additional tissue sampling. The use of a coaxial system facilitates the reinsertion of the biopsy needle at a tradeoff of increased cost and limitations in redirecting the needle.

When subtle calcifications are visualized as echogenic foci without a mass, it is critical that the first pass of the biopsy needle is well planned and well executed. After the first pass, a combination

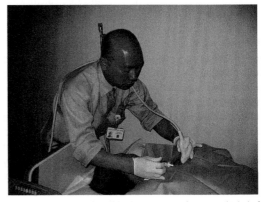

Fig. 5. Ultrasound-guided biopsy of a medial left breast lesion is performed by a right-handed operator standing at the level of the patient's head.

of air, blood, and fluid may obscure the target, and subsequent passes may be performed less optimally. Thus, vacuum-assisted biopsy devices are generally preferred for sampling calcifications. Vacuum-assisted biopsy devices are currently available as 14- to 8-gauge systems. Based on experience in stereotactic breast biopsy, vacuum-assisted biopsy devices represent a significant improvement in the accuracy of percutaneous imaged-guided biopsy of breast calcifications, compared with automated core biopsy needles. Vacuum-assisted biopsy devices are usually inserted once with sonographic guidance and are placed under the targeted lesion, and multiple samples can be obtained. The current use of 8- and 9-gauge vacuum-assisted biopsy devices generates larger samples, resulting in the retrieval of larger volumes of tissues in a shorter time.

The targeted lesion has to be placed exactly along the projected line of needle advancement with automated core biopsy needles. Vacuum-assisted biopsy devices allow the operator greater maneuvering capabilities, as the targeted lesion can be approached from a greater distance, with the probe placed below the targeted lesion. The placement of the skin incision for needle insertion depends on the depth of the targeted lesion. For most lesions, the skin incision is placed 1 cm from the edge of the transducer. Skin incisions located more than 2 to 3 cm from the transducer may be required if the targeted lesion is located close to the chest wall. This approach will facilitate the needle to be nearly horizontal. Thus, the needle can be advanced in a safe manner. This technique is especially important when automated core biopsy needles are used. The skin and the subcutaneous tissues are lifted when the skin incision is made. This maneuver improves the ease of insertion of larger vacuum-assisted biopsy devices. Visualization of the entire biopsy needle is optimal when the needle is nearly horizontal along the transducer's focal plane.

Ultrasound-guided breast biopsy procedures are highly operator dependent, and require good eye-hand coordination and the ability to navigate 3-dimensionally. Ultrasound-guided biopsy of breast calcifications without associated masses can be challenging, even for experienced operators. It is important that specimen radiographs are obtained to confirm the presence of calcifications at the end of the biopsy procedure. A clip marker is then placed to document the biopsy site. Clip placement is needed especially in small lesions following vacuum-assisted biopsy and after biopsy of highly suspicious large lesions that will likely be treated with neoadjuvant chemotherapy. Different types of clips should be considered when there is more than one targeted lesion. If the targeted lesion is highly suspicious and the need for breast MRI to determine the extent of disease is likely, clips with minimal MRI susceptibility artifacts should be considered. Post-biopsy mammograms are then obtained to document proper clip placement.

The most crucial next step after an ultrasound-guided biopsy is the correlation of the pathology results with the imaging findings. As discussed earlier, the radiologist performing the biopsy should independently assess the targeted lesion's probability of malignancy before the procedure to appropriately choose the method of biopsy and to determine what biopsy instrument will be used. When the pathologic diagnosis is rendered, a review of all available imaging studies is performed to ensure that the pathology results are concordant with the imaging findings. The pathology reports should include the presence or the absence of the targeted calcifications. The presence of calcifications does not necessarily mean that the sampling has been adequate, but the absence of calcifications requires an additional procedure: either repeat percutaneous biopsy or surgical excision.

If the lesions are placed appropriately in BI-RADS categories 3, 4a, and 4b, a benign histologic diagnosis is expected. Follow-up imaging is usually scheduled in 6 months in cases with concordant benign results. When a lesion is assessed to be BI-RADS 5 (highly suggestive of malignancy), a malignant result is expected. Therefore, a benign histologic diagnosis for a BI-RADS 5 lesion is considered discordant, and repeat percutaneous biopsy or surgical excision should be performed. Lesions placed in BI-RADS 4c (50% chance of malignancy) present a management conundrum when the pathology results are benign. When the lesions are prospectively and appropriately assessed as BI-RADS 4c, a larger biopsy device should be employed and a larger number of specimens should be obtained.

The larger vacuum-assisted biopsy devices allow the possibility of removal of the entire sonographically visible lesion. Parker and colleagues[14] performed 124 sonographically guided breast biopsies in 113 patients using an 11-gauge vacuum-assisted biopsy device. All lesions were 1.5 cm or less in greatest dimension. Sonography and mammography after biopsy showed that 88% (110 of 124 lesions) had no imaging evidence of the targeted lesion. There were 19 invasive cancers, 1 case of DCIS, 3 cases of atypical ductal hyperplasia (ADH), 1 case of atypical lobular hyperplasia (ALH), and 1 phyllodes tumor. There was no underestimation of disease. One invasive cancer was entirely removed by the vacuum-assisted biopsy device. Follow-up imaging in 6 months may be appropriate for benign lesions that have been adequately sampled. If there is a possibility of inadequate sampling, a repeat percutaneous biopsy or a surgical excision is recommended. The increased use of vacuum-assisted biopsy devices has improved the diagnostic accuracy of percutaneous sampling of breast calcifications.

The diagnosis of high-risks lesions such as ADH, lobular carcinoma in situ (LCIS), radial scar, and mucinous lesions on imaging-guided percutaneous biopsy warrants surgical excision. As discussed earlier, the underestimation rate is significantly higher with 14 gauge automated spring-loaded cutting needles compared with 14 gauge vacuum-assisted biopsy devices and 11-gauge vacuum-assisted biopsy devices.[6–9,15–17]

Lourenco and colleagues[16] performed a retrospective review of 1223 consecutive stereotactic vacuum-assisted breast biopsies and found no significant difference between 11-gauge biopsy and 9-gauge biopsy in underestimation of ADH and DCIS. In the 11-gauge biopsy group, 13 of 46 (28%) of ADH were upgraded to 12 DCIS and 1 invasive carcinoma; 35 of 122 (29%) cases of DCIS were upgraded to invasive cancers. In the 9-gauge biopsy group, 8 of 27 (29%) ADH were upgraded to 6 DCIS and 2 invasive cancers; 10 of 44 (23%) cases of DCIS were upgraded to invasive cancers.

SUMMARY

At present, suspicious and highly suspicious breast calcifications are usually biopsied under stereotactic guidance. Ultrasonography can be performed in patients with highly suspicious calcifications and dense fibroglandular tissues to identify an associated sonographically visible mass. In cases of calcifications associated with a sonographically visible mass, ultrasound-guided biopsy can decrease the underestimation rate. Improved resolution with current state-of-the-art equipment allows the possibility of ultrasound-guided biopsy of calcifications without a sonographically visible mass, and may provide an alternative approach in cases that are not amenable to stereotactic biopsy.

REFERENCES

1. D'Orsi CJ, Bassett LW, Berg WA, et al. BI-RADS mammography. In: D'Orsi CJ, Mendelson EB, Ikeda DM, et al, editors. Breast Imaging Reporting and Data System: ACR BI-RADS—breast imaging atlas. 4th edition. Reston (VA): American College of Radiology; 2003. p. 61–128.
2. Li CI, Daling JR. Changes in breast cancer incidence rates in the United States by histologic subtype and race/ethnicity 1995 to 2004. Cancer Epidemiol Biomarkers Prev 2007;16:2773–80.
3. Feig SA, Yaffe MJ. Digital mammography, computer-aided diagnosis, and telemammography. Radiol Clin North Am 1995;33:1205–30.
4. Liberman L, Abramson AF, Squires FB, et al. The breast imaging reporting and data system: positive predictive value of mammographic features and final assessment categories. AJR Am J Roentgenol 1998;171:35–40.
5. Burnside ES, Ochsner JE, Fowler KJ, et al. Use of microcalcification descriptors in BI-RADS 4th edition to stratify risk of malignancy. Radiology 2007;242:388–95.
6. Jackman RJ, Nowels KW, Rodriguez-Soto J, et al. Stereotactic, automated, large-core needle biopsy of nonpalpable breast lesions: false-negative and histologic underestimation rates after long-term follow-up. Radiology 1999;210:799–805.
7. Liberman L, Smolkin JH, Dershaw DD, et al. Calcifications retrieval at stereotactic, 11-gauge, directional, vacuum-assisted breast biopsy. Radiology 1998;208:251–60.
8. Liberman L, Gougoutas CA, Zakowski MF, et al. Calcifications highly suggestive of malignancy: comparison of breast biopsy methods. AJR Am J Roentgenol 2001;177:165–72.
9. Eby PR, Ochsner JE, DeMartini WB, et al. Frequency and upgrade rates of atypical ductal hyperplasia diagnosed at stereotactic vacuum-assisted breast biopsy: 9- versus 11-gauge. AJR Am J Roentgenol 2009;192:229–34.
10. Yang WT, Suen M, Ahuja A, et al. In vivo demonstration of microcalcification in breast cancer using high resolution ultrasound. Br J Radiol 1997;70:685–90.
11. Moon WK, Im JG, Koh YH, et al. US of mammographically detected clustered microcalcifications. Radiology 2000;217:849–54.
12. Hashimoto BE. Sonography of ductal carcinoma in situ. Ultrasound Clin 2006;1:631–43.
13. Soo MS, Baker JA, Rosen EL. Sonographic detection and sonographically guided biopsy of breast microcalcifications. AJR Am J Roentgenol 2003;180:941–8.
14. Parker SH, Klaus AJ, McWey PJ, et al. Sonographically guided directional vacuum-assisted breast biopsy using a handheld device. AJR Am J Roentgenol 2001;177:405–8.
15. Burbank F. Stereotactic breast biopsy of atypical ductal hyperplasia and ductal carcinoma in situ lesions: improved accuracy with directional, vacuum-assisted biopsy. Radiology 1997;202:843–7.

16. Lourenco AP, Mainiero MB, Lazarus E, et al. Stereo-tactic breast biopsy: comparison of histologic underestimation rates with 11- and 9-gauge vacuum-assisted breast biopsy. AJR Am J Roentgenol 2007;189:W275–9.

17. Kohr JR, Eby PR, Allison KH, et al. Risk of upgrade of atypical ductal hyperplasia after stereotactic breast biopsy: effects of number of foci and complete removal of calcifications. Radiology 2010;255: 723–30.

Ultrasound of Breast Implants and Soft Tissue Silicone

Michael P. McNamara Jr, MD[a,b,*],
Michael S. Middleton, MD, PhD[c]

KEYWORDS

• Ultrasound • Breast implants • Silicone

There are a wide variety of breast implant types (**Table 1**).[1] Most implants that are clinically encountered are single-lumen, saline-filled; single-lumen, silicone gel–filled; standard double-lumen (saline-filled outer, silicone gel-filled inner); and reverse double-lumen (silicone gel–filled outer, saline-filled inner). The reverse double-lumen type has been most frequently used in patients who have undergone reconstruction. Single-lumen, saline-filled and multilumen implants have valves to allow inflation with saline. Implant shells are made of a silicone elastomer rubber and vary in thickness from less than a millimeter to about 2 millimeters. The outer shell surface can be smooth or textured (fine or coarse) and polyurethane coating has been used for some implants (eg, Même, Replicon, and some implants manufactured outside the United States). Almost all implant shells are formed on a mushroom-shaped mandrel and thus have a several-centimeter hole in the back that is closed late in manufacturing with a shell patch (a round sheet of usually thicker silicone elastomer bonded or affixed to the implant shell with a silicone glue). Silicone gel–filled implants are filled via a needle usually placed through the shell patch, with the tiny hole closed with a small drop of silicone glue.

Sponge implants (usually Ivalon or Etheron) are occasionally encountered in older patients implanted before the introduction in 1963 of silicone gel–filled implants.

Although there was a moratorium on the sale of silicone gel–filled breast implants for augmentation in the United States beginning in 1992, silicone gel–filled implants remained available for reconstruction and revision surgery through adjunct study protocols. Manufacturers were required to initiate safety and efficacy trials and submit a Pre–Market Approval Application (PMA). In November, 2006 the US Food and Drug Administration approved the sale of silicone gel–filled implants for augmentation and reconstruction in the United States from 2 manufacturers: Inamed (now owned by Allergan) and Mentor.[2]

Although not marketed or sold in the United States, silicone gel–containing implants are produced for international use by other manufacturers such as Eurosilicone in France and Nagor in the United Kingdom. Another manufacturer, Poly Implants Prothese of France, encountered regulatory issues and went into receivership in March 2010.[3]

Breast implants can be placed via inframammary, periareolar, or axillary incisions and most commonly reside in a subglandular (prepectoral) or submuscular (subpectoral, beneath pectoralis major) position. In the latter, the inferior margin of pectoralis major is generally left unattached.

Implants are more or less underfilled (with silicone gel, saline, or both). Placement within the body results in the surface of the implant invaginating, resulting in folds that can show a variable, often undulating, appearance on imaging. All

[a] Breast Imaging and Intervention, Department of Radiology, Case School of Medicine, MetroHealth Medical Center, MH-2500, MetroHealth Boulevard, Cleveland, OH 44109, USA
[b] Uniformed Services, University of the Health Sciences, Bethesda, MD, USA
[c] Department of Radiology, University of California, San Diego, CA, USA
* Corresponding author. Breast Imaging and Intervention, Department of Radiology, Case School of Medicine, MetroHealth Medical Center, MH-2500, MetroHealth Boulevard, Cleveland, OH 44109.
E-mail address: mmcnamara@metrohealth.org

Ultrasound Clin 6 (2011) 345–368
doi:10.1016/j.cult.2011.05.002
1556-858X/11/$ – see front matter © 2011 Published by Elsevier Inc.

Table 1
Implant types

Implant Type	Description	Frequency (%)[a]
1. Single lumen, silicone gel filled	Silicone gel filled	79.62
2. Single lumen, adjustable	Silicone gel filled, to which a variable amount of saline could be added at time of placement	0.85
3. Saline, dextran, or PVP	Dextran-filled (some early implants), PVP-filled (Bioplasty), and the rest saline filled	6.23
4. Standard double lumen	Silicone gel inner lumen, saline outer lumen	11.12
5. Reverse double lumen	Saline inner lumen, silicone gel outer lumen	0.48
6. Reverse adjustable double lumen	Silicone gel inner and outer lumens, variable amount of saline added to inner lumen at time of placement	0.22
7. Gel-gel double lumen	Silicone gel inner and outer lumens	0.05
8. Triple lumen	Silicone gel inner and middle lumens, saline outer lumen	0.42
9. Cavon	Cohesive silicone gel, no shell	0.15
10. Custom	Nonstandard implant type, size, shape, fill (individualized)	0.13
11. Pectus	Solid silicone elastomer pectoralis muscle replacement implant	0.05
12. Sponge	Ivalon, Etheron, polyethylene, plastic strips, and so forth (solid or hollow, simple or compound, some encased in plastic bag)	0.65
13. Sponge adjustable	Silicone elastomer shell (polyurethane coated), polyurethane sponge inside, dextran filled or saline filled	0.02
14. Other	Triglyceride, or fill other than noted earlier	0.00

Abbreviation: PVP, polyvinylpyrrolidone.
[a] Percentage of a cohort of 9966 implants evaluated at the University of California San Diego. In clinical ultrasound practice, the percentage of saline-filled breast implants is much higher. The percentages are provided here to offer insight into the rarity of the more unusual implants.
Adapted from Middleton MS, McNamara MP Jr. Breast implant classification with MR imaging correlation. Radiographics 2000;20:E1.

implants are surrounded by a soft tissue, biologic, fibrous capsule, often within weeks of implantation (**Fig. 1**).

Independent of implant integrity, the fibrous capsule may thicken and contract considerably over time and may calcify (or even ossify) (**Fig. 2**). Calcification is generally not seen for approximately 10 years, but contraction of the fibrous capsule, which occurs more frequently, is variable in onset. Capsular contracture/calcification of the fibrous capsule implies nothing about implant integrity. When a silicone gel–filled implant ruptures, the fibrous capsule tends to contain the gel (grossly maintaining the clinically apparent form of the implant) unless it, too, is breeched. Rupture of a silicone gel–filled implant can result in progressive collapse, generally gradual, of the shell so that the shell is in the gel rather than the gel being in the shell. The sequence of uncollapsed to minimally collapsed, partially collapsed, and fully collapsed rupture is illustrated, from a sonographer's viewpoint, in **Fig. 3**.

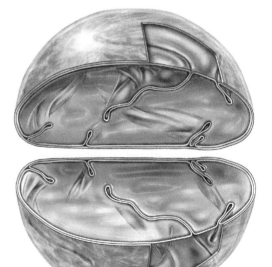

Fig. 1. A single-lumen implant. The surrounding fibrous capsule is shown with a cutaway to show the origin of several of the folds.

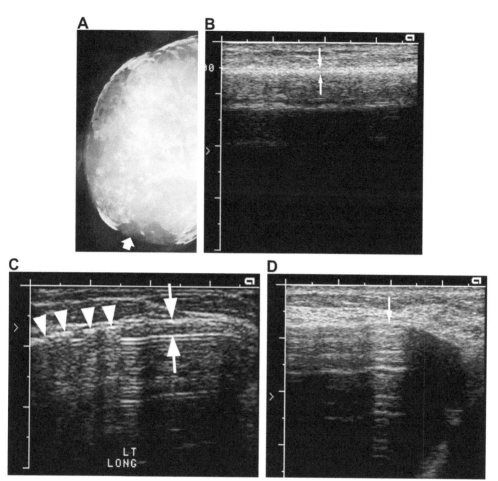

Fig. 2. Calcification of the fibrous capsule. (*A*) Mammogram of a sponge implant showing heavy calcification of the fibrous capsule. Mammographically, sponges are of lower density than silicone gel and higher in density than saline, and do not have a shell (*arrow*). For silicone gel–containing implants, gaps in the calcification of a fibrous capsule may be used as acoustic windows. (*B*) Calcification of the fibrous capsule of a single-lumen silicone gel–filled implant resulting in a fuzzy appearance of the capsule (*arrows*), a typical appearance. The resultant complex reverberations in the near field of the implant prevented identification of rupture of this implant, known to be present by magnetic resonance imaging. (*C*) Another silicone gel–filled implant. Calcification of the fibrous capsule is indicated by the arrowheads. At a gap in the calcification where the capsule is not calcified, evidence of rupture can be seen, as indicated by the arrows (see drop-away sign later). (*D*) Another silicone gel–filled implant with a fuzzy-capsule sign. At times, the calcification is thick and can even proceed to ossification with a prominent ring-down artifact (*arrow*).

This article provides the sonographer and sonologist with an overview of normal and abnormal implant findings, reviews the spectrum of appearance of soft tissue silicone, and discusses some pitfalls that can be encountered.

IMAGING EVALUATION

Although use of the modality has evolved with time, magnetic resonance (MR) imaging has become the generally preferred modality for evaluating the integrity of silicone gel–filled breast implants.[4–17]

Nevertheless, patients with implants are frequently encountered in the practice of breast sonography.

Most often, the patient with implants presents for evaluation of a clinical breast parenchymal problem or mammographic finding that is unrelated to the implants, and images may incidentally contain portions of implant. In this setting, unless a dedicated set of images has been acquired tailored to evaluate implants, it is appropriate, and prudent, to state in the ultrasound report that this study is not a dedicated evaluation of the patient's implant(s), because technical factors that are optimized to visualize breast parenchyma

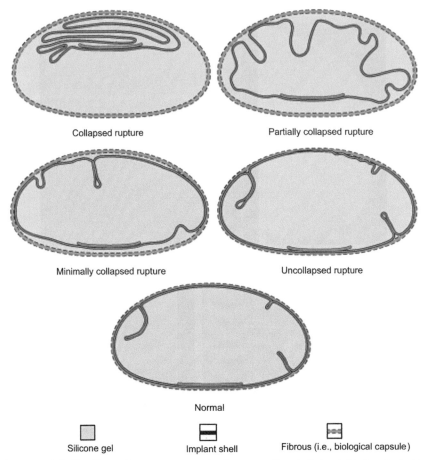

Fig. 3. The degrees of shell collapse from a sonographer's perspective. Left to right, top to bottom: collapsed rupture, partially collapsed rupture, minimally collapsed rupture, uncollapsed rupture, and, at the bottom, the normal appearance for comparison.

are generally suboptimal for implant evaluation. If there is an unequivocal or suspicious implant-related finding that is incidentally included on any of the images, judicious, limited comment may be offered in the report with the suggestion of proceeding with additional directed imaging as appropriate.

Occasionally, patients are referred for assessment of the location and extent of soft tissue silicone and, when MR imaging is not feasible or is contraindicated, determination of the integrity of a silicone gel–containing implant.

In the literature, sonography has been shown to have value in implant evaluation and detection of the presence and extent of soft tissue silicone.[7,15,17–30] Identifying the classic stepladder sign, also known as the wavy-line sign and linguine sign, is useful for identification of collapsed rupture.

We have found that ultrasound offers overlapping and complementary diagnostic capabilities (Table 2).[15] MR imaging is superior in showing the signs of all stages of collapse of ruptured silicone gel–filled implants, evaluating patients with heavy calcification of the fibrous capsule, and studying unusual implants. Sonography can identify some cases of uncollapsed rupture and many cases of partially and fully collapsed rupture. Uncollapsed rupture cannot be excluded sonographically or with MR imaging, but MR imaging is unequivocally better in this setting.

When an implant is primarily studied with ultrasound, if there is uncertainty as to the reliability of the findings, MR evaluation should be considered, if possible.

In our experience, sonography is more sensitive than MR imaging in identifying the presence and extent of smaller amounts of soft tissue silicone. Sonography has the additional advantage of being less costly, requiring less imaging time, and entailing less discomfort for the patient.

Neither MR imaging nor sonography, is needed for primary evaluation of single-lumen, saline-filled

Table 2
MR imaging versus ultrasound (US) for implant evaluation

	US	MR Imaging
Uncollapsed rupture	+	++++
Minimally collapsed rupture	++	++++
Partially collapsed rupture	+++	++++
Complete collapsed rupture	++++	++++
Implant evaluation in patients with calcified fibrous capsules	+	++++
Evaluation of uncommon or unusual appearing implants	+	++++
Silicone granuloma	++++	+++
Silicone gel cysts	++++	++++
Silicone adenopathy	++++	++
Time required for evaluation	++++	++
Cost	++++	+
Patient comfort	++++	++
Learning curve speed and ease	++	++++

Abbreviation: +, relative strengths/weaknesses of the modalities contrasted and compared.

implants. Unlike rupture of a silicone gel–filled implant, where the fibrous capsule often acts to maintain the overall shape and form of the implant, saline lost from an implant is absorbed by/through the fibrous capsule so loss of volume of the device occurs. This loss of volume is almost always apparent to the patient and her physician.

Sonography may be obtained if infection or bleeding-related complications requiring imaging are suspected.

CLINICAL HISTORY

Irrespective of whether a patient has been referred for a breast parenchymal problem, or for primary evaluation of an implant or of soft tissue silicone, we recommend obtaining implant-related history. Because it is common for a patient to have had more than 1 implant, on either or both sides, we seek information regarding the current/prior implant type(s), dates of surgeries, the status of prior implants on explantation (intact or ruptured), any known history of residual soft tissue silicone, as well as the current clinical issue/complaint/finding that needs to be evaluated. Clinical information is usually helpful and is occasionally crucial, so it is important to actively solicit.

Obtaining clinical information frequently is a challenge for the imager. However, at the time of surgery, the type of implant is usually recorded within the operative note and often a copy of the tags (stickers that provide technical data about the implant manufacturer, style, catalog or product number, and lot number) is given to the patient (**Fig. 4**). Many patients are happy to provide this data. If not known or evident from prior imaging, the product/catalog number on the tags can be searched for on the Internet or by looking them up in a catalog to determine the implant type.[15] When implant type is known, deviation from the expected imaging appearance of that implant type may be more readily appreciated. Because the normal appearance of certain types of implants can be confusing, and can simulate the appearance of rupture, knowledge of implant type can minimize the likelihood of diagnostic error.

TECHNICAL APPROACH TO SCANNING

The patient is placed in what we term the standard position: supine and turned to the contralateral side sufficiently so that the breast/implant flattens as evenly as possible against the chest wall (**Fig. 5**). The ipsilateral arm is superiorly abducted, with the elbow flexed. To facilitate comfortable positioning, a positioning wedge or rolled sheet is placed laterally under the ipsilateral thorax, flank, and hips, and a rolled towel is placed for arm support.

Unless absolutely necessary, we do not have the patient's head on a pillow, because the supraclavicular region is also scanned to look for evidence of adenopathy.

First, we sweep the peripheral edge of the implant from 12:00 around the device until we again reach 12:00. The transducer is oriented radially and centered so that the junction of the edge of the implant and adjacent soft tissues can be searched for evidence of extrusions/soft tissue silicone. Most often, soft tissue silicone from current or prior rupture is in immediate proximity to the implant, usually at this interface. Care must be taken not to apply too much pressure, because some smaller direct extrusions can be flattened or reduced in volume and become less apparent.

Next, we insonate the anterior aspect of the implant with the transducer oriented transversely and sweep cephalically to caudally with overlapping passes progressing from medial to lateral so that the entirety of the implant is studied. Care is taken to adjust the angle of insonation and center the transducer so that the beam is directed perpendicular to the shell/inner surface of the fibrous capsule. In this way, we optimize our ability to obtain specular reflections from the shell. During these passes, we look for sonographic

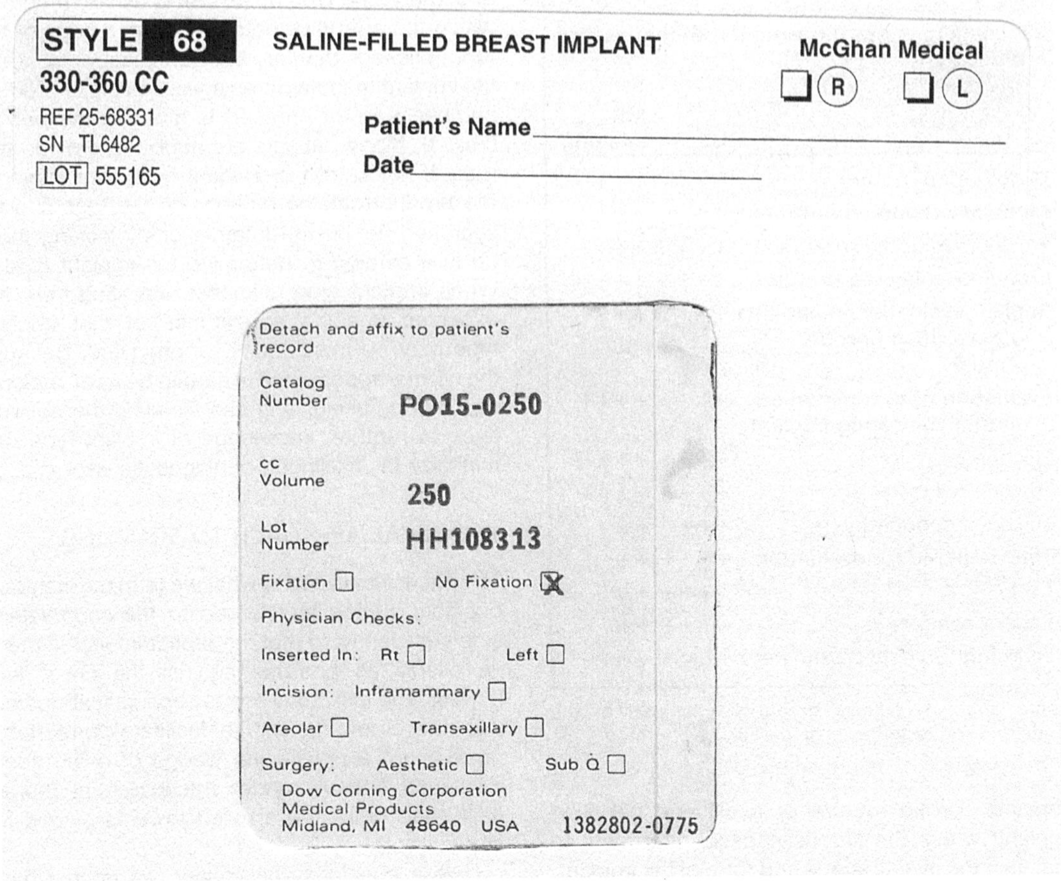

STYLE **68**   SALINE-FILLED BREAST IMPLANT   McGhan Medical
☐ R   ☐ L

330-360 CC
REF 25-68331
SN TL6482
LOT 555165

Patient's Name_____

Date_____

Detach and affix to patient's record

Catalog Number   **PO15-0250**

cc Volume   **250**

Lot Number   **HH108313**

Fixation ☐   No Fixation ☒

Physician Checks:

Inserted In: Rt ☐   Left ☐

Incision: Inframammary ☐

Areolar ☐   Transaxillary ☐

Surgery: Aesthetic ☐   Sub Q ☐

Dow Corning Corporation
Medical Products
Midland, MI 48640 USA   1382802-0775

Fig. 4. Implant tags. Style, catalog, and product numbers allow the original construction of the implant to be determined.

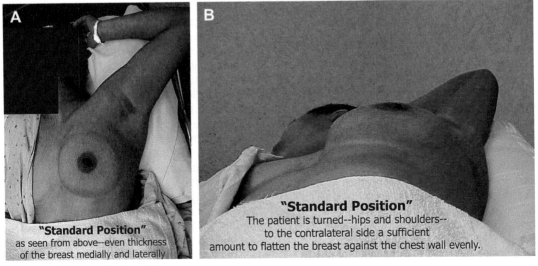

A

"Standard Position"
as seen from above--even thickness
of the breast medially and laterally

B

"Standard Position"
The patient is turned--hips and shoulders--
to the contralateral side a sufficient
amount to flatten the breast against the chest wall evenly.

Fig. 5. (*A, B*) The standard position.

signs of implant integrity or rupture. The focal zones are adjusted so that they are at the level of the inner surface of the fibrous capsule/within the first centimeter or so of the implant.

The soft tissues of the anterior thorax are then examined from the level of the clavicle to below the inframammary fold and from midsternum to midaxillary line with the same overlapping transverse imaging, with the focal zones set anterior to the implant, appropriate for searching for silicone within soft tissue planes and parenchyma.

Next, we survey the lymphatic drainage pathways of the breast (**Fig. 6**). Axillary level 1 (lateral to the edge of the pectoralis minor muscle) is studied with overlapping transverse passes of the transducer, using firm pressure. Axillary level 2 (deep to pectoralis minor, above and below the subclavian vessels) and axillary level 3 (medial to pectoralis minor) are studied with the transducer oriented longitudinally, just inferior to the clavicle, from medial to lateral and then with the probe oriented transversely. Rotter nodes (between pectoralis major and minor) are sought with the transducer oriented transversely. Most pathologic Rotter nodes are immediately contiguous to the small vessels that run cephalocaudad between the muscles near the midpoint, from medial to lateral, of pectoralis minor. The nodes of the internal mammary chain are contiguous to the sternum medial, between or lateral to the internal mammary artery and vein(s). When notable, supraclavicular nodes are generally more medial than lateral. Insonation of the internal mammary chain

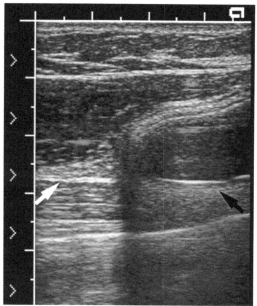

Fig. 7. Long-axis ultrasound image, oriented parallel to the chest wall, of a single-lumen, saline-filled, textured-surface implant (McGhan Biocell). The implant is submuscular in location between pectoralis major and pectoralis minor. Imaging was facilitated by adducting the patient's ipsilateral arm to her side. The arrows indicate the anterior chest wall; the anterior aspect of pectoralis minor. Note that fine muscle detail deep to the implant is obscured by reverberations from the heavy texturing of the implant shell.

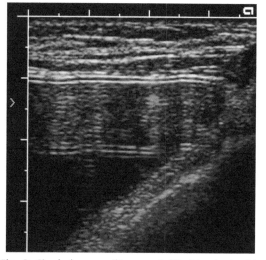

Fig. 8. Single-lumen, silicone gel–filled implant with a smooth surface. The shell is seen as 2 parallel lines. The outer aspect of the shell blends imperceptivity with the inner surface of the fibrous capsule. The reverberations in the near field are a normal, expected finding.

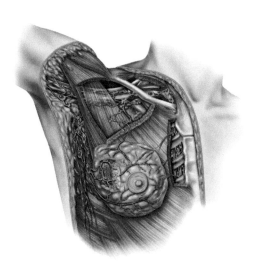

Fig. 6. The major lymphatic drainage pathways of the breast. Axillary nodes are divided into level 1, 2, and 3 (see text).

and supraclavicular region is done both longitudinally and transversely.

If any disorder is noted, images are recorded both transversely and longitudinally with the appropriate measurements annotated on, and then removed from, the images.

If an implant is deemed likely to be intact and there is no adenopathy, we take a single image of each quadrant (showing intimate application of the shell to the inner surface of the fibrous capsule).

A longitudinal/radial image is then obtained at the cephalic margin of the implant (generally somewhere from the 11:00 to 1:00 region). The image is optimized technically to show whether the implant is subglandular or subpectoral/submuscular in location and to allow information regarding the contents (silicone gel or saline) of 1 or more of the shell(s) to be deduced. The depth of field for the longitudinal/radial image should be adjusted so that the chest wall is visualized. The junction of

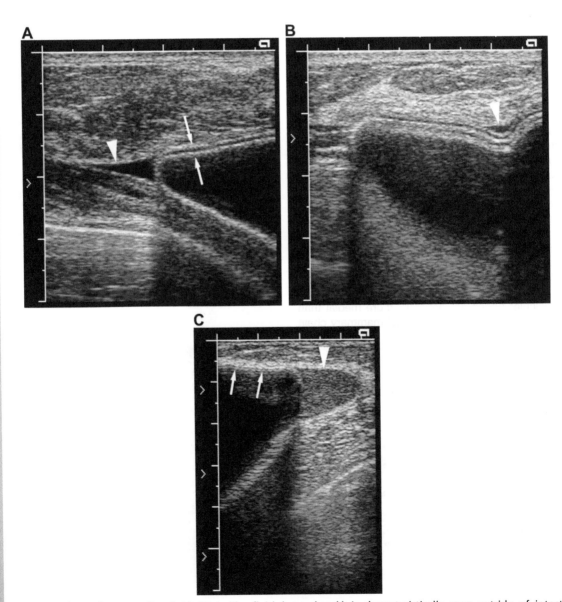

Fig. 9. Subcapsular waterlike fluid. Waterlike fluid (*arrowheads*) is characteristically seen outside of intact textured-surface (*A*) and (*B*) as well as polyurethane-coated implants (*C*). The fluid seen with the latter typically contains echogenic particles, believed to be denuded polyurethane. Where subcapsular waterlike fluid is present, the inner surface of the fibrous capsule can be seen separate from the outer surface of the implant shell. Usually, the margin of the capsule is angular, as in (*A*) (*arrows*). The rounded appearance seen in (*C*) is unusual and probably related to the large amount of subcapsular waterlike fluid present in this case (*arrows*).

the implant and the superior soft tissues should be centered within the image and the angle of insonation adjusted so that the transducer is as parallel as possible to the chest wall (**Fig. 7**). At times, acquisition of this image can be facilitated by having the patient place her arm down at her side.

Assuming no disorder is noted, a single transverse image of the level 1 axilla is recorded, indicating that the lymphatic drainage tracts have been examined.

THE NORMAL SONOGRAPHIC APPEARANCE OF BREAST IMPLANTS

The normal appearance, overall, varies by implant type and style.

Regardless of implant type and whether it is intact or ruptured, the most important information is in the implant's sonographic near field (ie, within the first centimeter or so deep to the fibrous capsule), as illustrated in **Fig. 3**. Although it is common to have near-field reverberation artifact within the implant, its distracting effect can generally be minimized when the time/gain compensation curve and overall gain are adjusted and subtle adjustments to the angulation of the transducer are made to ensure that specular reflections are obtained from the shell. Assuming that there is no obscuration by calcification of the fibrous capsule, details regarding the implant shell(s) can usually be seen.

Paradoxically, in imaging implants, less is more. We almost always restrict imaging of the implant itself to its near field (at most the anterior half). This technique results in more pixels of the image devoted to where signs of likely intactness or rupture can best be seen. The findings are larger on the monitor, and images and subtle details are easier to appreciate. Conversely, if the field of view is enlarged to include the posterior wall of the implant, the relevant details in the near field are more difficult to see and can easily be overlooked, because they can be subtle. Visualization of the posterior half of the implant and chest wall posterior to the implant are necessary in only 2 circumstances: (1) the routine image done from 11:00 to 1:00, and (2) in the rare instance in which it is necessary to search for a valve posteriorly. In the former, the relationship of the superior aspect of the implant to the underlying chest wall is of interest. The image provides information regarding the implant type and anatomic location, as noted earlier. In the latter, occasionally an implant rotates or is intentionally be placed so that the shell patch is anterior and, in a single-lumen saline-filled device, the valve may be posterior.

Silicone gel, as well as saline, is usually anechoic. Although echogenic gel can be seen in the setting of

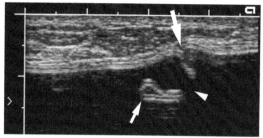

Fig. 10. Normal fold of a single-lumen implant with a finely textured surface. A small amount of waterlike fluid can be seen in the tip of the fold (the inner, textured surface of the fold is the outside of the implant shell and the fluid is, technically, subcapsular in location) (*arrows*).

a failed/ruptured implant, it can also be seen in an intact implant and should never be used as a sign of rupture, in and of itself. We have seen echogenic gel (from nearly anechoic to very echogenic) as an idiopathic finding in single-lumen, silicone gel–filled implants as well as in single-lumen, silicone gel/saline implants and in the setting of barrier disruption (discussed later). When silicone gel in a lumen is echogenic, the shell and folds can still be seen because specular reflections from implant elastomer shell are always brighter than from silicone gel.

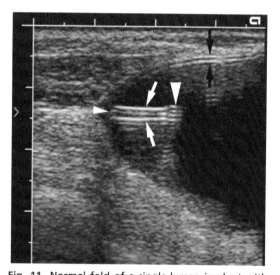

Fig. 11. Normal fold of a single-lumen implant with a smooth surface. The interface of the apposing (outer) shell surfaces forming the fold merge into a single line sonographically (*small arrowhead*) and the inner surfaces of the fold are generally better seen (*small white arrows*). At the tip of the fold (*large arrowhead*), the outer edges of the shell (the inner surfaces of the tip) are typically slightly separated. Because it is made of 2 layers, the fold is twice the thickness of the shell (*small black arrows*).

The key feature to actively look for while scanning is apposition of the implant shell to the inner surface of the fibrous capsule.

Except at the base of folds, when an implant is intact the shell is seen as 1 or more echogenic parallel lines immediately deep to the inner surface of the fibrous capsule (**Fig. 8**).

Unless grossly thickened or calcified, the outer surface of the fibrous capsule is generally indistinguishable from the surrounding soft tissue superficial to it.

When an implant is intact, the inner surface of the fibrous capsule is often difficult to see as a distinct entity because it tends to blend acoustically with the outer surface of the shell.

The inner surface of the fibrous capsule can most easily be seen with intact textured and polyurethane-coated implants because some waterlike fluid is commonly present between the fibrous capsule and outer aspect of the implant shell. This subcapsular fluid can be seen at the edge of the implant and at the base of folds, particularly shallow folds, and should not be confused with silicone outside of the implant shell (**Fig. 9**). The base of a fold is often V-shaped and may be seen if a fold originates from the anterior surface of the implant (**Fig. 10**). If the fold arises more laterally, refraction artifact generally prevents the base from being seen clearly (**Fig. 11**). Folds are generally difficult or impossible to visualize in their

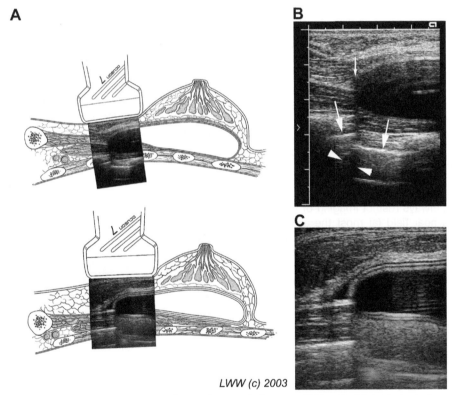

LWW (c) 2003

Fig. 12. Translation artifact. (*A*) Diagram with superimposed ultrasound images of intact, single-lumen, silicone gel–filled implants. The implant in the upper image is submuscular and has a smooth shell. The implant in the lower image is subglandular and textured. In both images, the structures deep to the implant are artifactually displaced posteriorly, because the implants are gel filled. (*B*) The longitudinal ultrasound image used in the upper diagram in (*A*). Translation artifact displaces the apparent location of the soft tissues deep to the implant posteriorly. This displacement is most easily appreciated as the result of its effect on the pleural reflection (*large arrows*), which is continuous and linear in reality. Edge shadowing is seen at the margin of the implant (*small arrow*). Additional refraction artifact (*arrowheads*) is seen deep to the artifactual edge of the pleural margin. (*C*) The longitudinal ultrasound image used in the lower diagram in (*A*). The translation artifact is only deep to the silicone gel–containing lumen. There is a small amount of subcapsular waterlike fluid at the cephalic margin of the implant. This fluid is a normal finding with textured-surface implants and does not show the translation artifact, as expected, helping to distinguish it from silicone gel. Also note that there is snowstorm artifact deep to the implant: complex reverberations and refractions that are common deep to heavily textured implants and that should not be confused with silicone granuloma.

entirety with ultrasound. Given that they undulate and their position and orientation are not predictable, they can only rarely be imaged sufficiently parallel to the transducer face to be well seen.

There are some specific sonographic features that can help distinguish between implant types.

Single-lumen, Silicone Gel–filled versus Single-lumen, Saline-filled

The longitudinal/radial image obtained at the cephalic margin of the implant (generally somewhere from the 11:00 to 1:00 region) can be used to infer the type of material in the implant. Immediately deep to a silicone gel–filled lumen, the soft tissue plane appears to be displaced posteriorly,

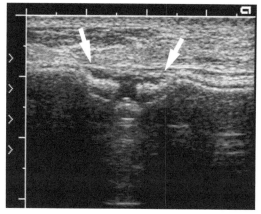

Fig. 13. Diaphragm valve (*arrows*).

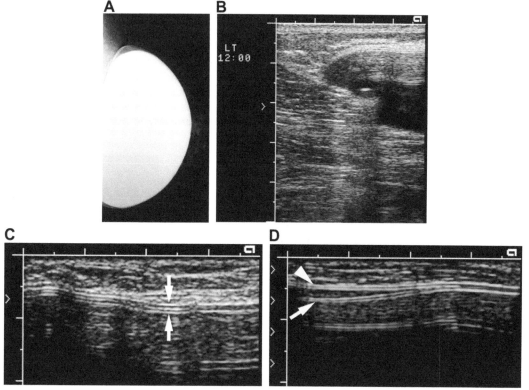

Fig. 14. Intact standard, double-lumen (saline-filled outer/silicone gel–filled inner) implants. (*A*) Mediolateral-oblique film-screen mammogram. At the superior aspect of the implant, and, to a lesser degree, at its inferior margin, the outer saline-containing lumen can be seen. The saline within that lumen is less dense than silicone, allowing both the inner and outer margins of the outer shell to be seen. (*B*) Longitudinal ultrasound of an intact subglandular, standard, double-lumen implant showing a translation artifact deep to the silicone gel–containing lumen and lack of translation deep to the saline-containing lumen. (*C*) Anterior aspect of a standard double lumen showing close apposition of both the inner and outer shells to the inner aspect of the fibrous capsule (*arrows*). Of the 3 parallel lines, the more superficial is a composite of the outer aspect of the outer shell and the inner surface of the fibrous capsule, the middle is the apposition of the inner surface of the outer shell and the outer surface of the inner shell, and the more posterior line is the inner aspect of the inner shell. Typically, there is a modest amount of saline in the outer lumen, so what fluid is seen is generally best seen at the superior margin of the implant, as in (*A*) and (*B*). (*D*) Anterior aspect of another standard double lumen near the superior edge; some fluid is seen between the outer and inner lumen shells (*arrows*); to the right of the image, the shells merge acoustically, as in (*C*).

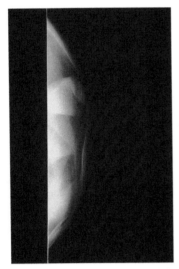

Fig. 15. Intact reverse double lumen (silicone gel–filled outer/saline-filled inner). The typical mammographic appearance is seen on an overpenetrated craniocaudal view.

a translation artifact, because the speed of sound in silicone gel is slower than in soft tissue. Because the ultrasound machine expects sound to be transmitted at approximately 1540 m/s, the slower transit time causes echoes deep to silicone gel to be displaced deeper than they really are. To clearly see this effect, it is important that the transducer be oriented parallel or nearly parallel to the chest wall (**Fig. 12**). The translation artifact also allows the subcapsular waterlike fluid to be distinguished from silicone gel.

When a saline-filled lumen is similarly insonated, the translation artifact is not seen: the echoes from the chest wall are linear and continuous both above and deep to the implant, as depicted in **Fig. 7**. Also, essentially all single-lumen, saline-filled implants have a fill valve, almost always anterior in location. There are various valve types, but the diaphragm valve is most common (**Fig. 13**).

Standard Double-lumen Implants

Standard double-lumen implants (saline-filled outer, silicone gel–filled inner) can have several appearances, depending on whether there is saline in the outer lumen and, if present, how much. The most straightforward way to determine that a standard

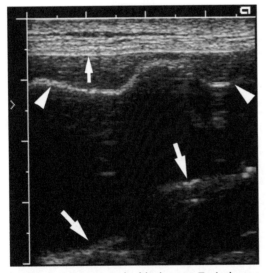

Fig. 16. Intact reverse double lumen. Typical sonographic appearance showing the characteristic thick, undulating, continuous line in the near field (*arrowheads*) that is the anterior interface between the outer and inner lumens. The anterior interface of the shells could be confused with a redundant fold. The distinction can be made by recognizing that the undulating interface does not terminate peripherally at the margin of the implant as a long, undulating fold can be expected to. The outer shell can be seen in contact with the fibrous capsule (*small arrow*), but is difficult to see, because the image is optimized to see the anterior interface. If the depth of field is sufficient, portions of the posterior interface of the shells may also be seen (*large arrows*).

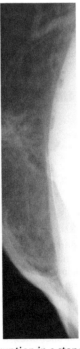

Fig. 17. Barrier disruption in a standard double-lumen implant. A salad-oil appearance is seen where there has been mixing of the silicone gel with the outer lumen saline. The device is still intact as a whole because the outer shell remains intact; this is best appreciated at the inferior aspect of the image.

double-lumen implant is intact is to show the saline in the outer lumen mammographically, focusing on the superior aspect of the implant on the mediolateral-oblique view (**Fig. 14A**). The corresponding appearance, taking advantage of the speed-of-sound translation artifact, can be seen sonographically when insonating at the 11:00 to 1:00 position (see **Fig. 14B**). The intact, standard, double-lumen implant is characterized by the outer shell being in intimate contact with the inner surface of the fibrous capsule. Because there is generally little to no saline present in the outer lumen anteriorly (at least when the patient is imaged with ultrasound and mammography), both the inner and outer shell may be intimately in contact with one another and the inner surface of the fibrous capsule, producing a triple-line sign (see **Fig. 14C, D**). If an intact outer lumen is shown mammographically or sonographically, the implant can be deemed effectively intact and no further imaging is necessary.

The mammographic appearance (on an overpenetrated film) of a reverse double-lumen (silicone gel–filled outer, saline-filled inner) implant is characteristic (**Fig. 15**). The amount of silicone gel in the outer lumen of this device is enough that it can be visualized sonographically anteriorly with the patient supine. When the device is intact the interface between the inner and outer lumen sonographically can be seen as a thick, undulating, continuous line in the implant's near field. When intact, the outer shell can be seen to be in intimate contact with the inner surface of the fibrous capsule. It is important to recognize and distinguish this appearance from the wavy-line or linguine sign of collapsed rupture. The typical and classic sonographic appearance of the reverse double-lumen is illustrated in **Fig. 16**.

IMPLANT FAILURE

Implant failure can occur in a variety of ways.

Deflation

Deflation refers to loss of volume from any saline-containing lumen of a breast implant, allowing saline to escape the device, as a whole. Usually, all or almost all of the saline escapes, and is absorbed by surrounding soft tissues. Deflation most commonly is caused by a tear or other defect in an (outer) implant shell but also can occur with fill-valve dysfunction. Deflation of a single-lumen, saline-filled implant results in breast volume loss, with resultant asymmetry usually apparent to patient and physician alike. Deflation of the outer lumen of a standard double-lumen implant may or may not be apparent because the volume of saline, relative to the amount of silicone gel, is

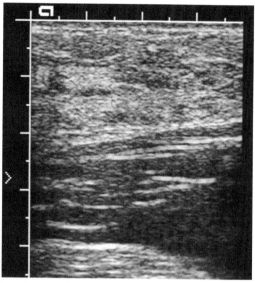

Fig. 18. Wavy-line sign (also known as the linguine or stepladder sign). The collapsed shell floating in the gel is seen sonographically as segments of single-layer thick shell (ie, not folds or outer/inner shells applied to one another, as in a reverse double lumen). Care must be taken to correlate with available history and other imaging studies, including mammograms, as noted earlier, because simulators of this appearance may be seen with intact (and ruptured) multilumen implants.

Table 3
University of California San Diego breast implant rupture results summary[a]

Implant Condition	Number of Implants (%)	
	Intracapsular	Extracapsular
No evidence of rupture	1095 (64.6)	NA
Indeterminate	130 (7.7)	0
Uncollapsed rupture	220 (13)	35 (2.1)
Minimally collapsed rupture	55 (3.2)	9 (0.5)
Partially collapsed rupture	7 (0.4)	14 (0.8)
Fully collapsed rupture	61 (3.6)	70 (4.1)

[a] Cohort of 1696 single-lumen, silicone gel–filled implants studied from 1992 to 1999.

Adapted from Middleton MS, McNamara MP. Breast implant imaging. Philadelphia: Lippincott Williams & Wilkins; 2003.

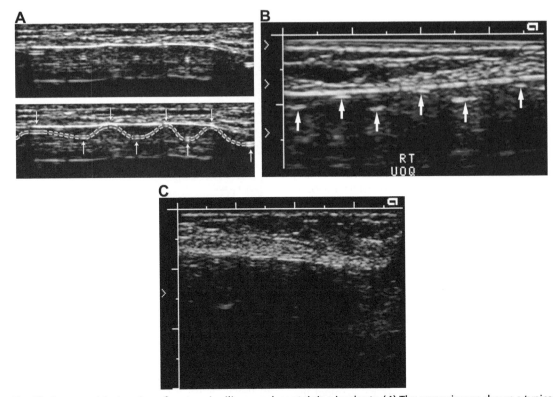

Fig. 19. Sonographic sine sign of rupture in silicone gel–containing implants. (*A*) The upper image shows a typical sine sign appearance: specular reflections occur only from the peaks and the troughs. The lower image shows the entire course of the shell diagrammatically. (*B*) The sine sign (*arrows*) in another patient. (*C*) Subtle sine sign in another patient is made more difficult to see because the depth of field is greater.

generally small. Deflation only of the outer lumen of a standard double-lumen implant, in the setting of an intact inner silicone gel–filled lumen, should not be termed rupture because the implant becomes, functionally, like an intact, single-lumen, silicone gel–filled implant, albeit of lower volume than when the implant was placed.

Barrier Disruption

Barrier disruption occurs when there is loss of integrity of only the shell separating silicone gel–filled and saline-filled lumens in a double-lumen or triple-lumen device, resulting in an admixture of silicone gel and saline. This admixture is sonographically difficult to detect directly, but the gel

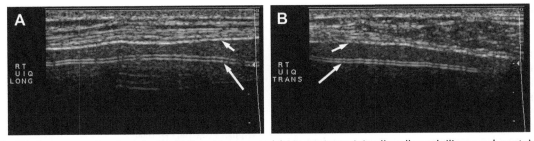

Fig. 20. Drop-away sign. Longitudinal (*A*) and transverse (*B*) images in a minimally collapsed silicone gel–containing rupture showing the shell (*long arrow*) displaced posteriorly from the inner surface of the fibrous capsule (*short arrow*) by a thick layer of silicone gel.

A   B

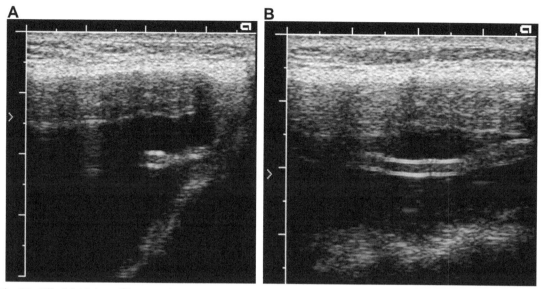

Fig. 21. Filled-fold sign. Silicone gel is within the tip of a fold, seen in short axis (*A*) and long axis (*B*). This sign is rarely seen and care must be taken not to confuse the filled-fold sign with the normal appearance of the fold in a textured implant, as seen in **Fig. 10.**

may be variably echogenic. It can be seen mammographically (**Fig. 17**). If the outer shell is intact, the implant is considered to be intact, as a whole, and becomes essentially like a single-lumen gel/saline implant (see **Table 1**).

Rupture

Rupture is best reserved for failure of the outer shell of a silicone gel–filled device, allowing silicone gel to escape the implant as whole. Unless there has been frank direct trauma, shells tend to fail from mechanical fatigue most often at the tip or base of a fold or at the edge of the shell patch. Silicone gel escapes the implant and, after some period of time, the implant shell may collapse as more and more gel becomes outside, rather than inside the implant. The MR imaging (and ultrasound) imaging appearance of ruptured implants varies from uncollapsed to minimally to partially to fully collapsed, as noted in **Fig. 3**. The defect in the shell (which varies from a microhole, difficult to see without a magnifying glass, to being many centimeters in size) is usually not seen on imaging and may be a challenge to find even when an explanted implant is examined.

The key to the diagnosis of rupture, both by imaging and by direct inspection by the surgeon or pathologist, is the presence of silicone gel on the outer surface of the (outer) implant shell. Silicone gel formally consists of a matrix of cross-linked long-chain silicone molecules, and free (or fluid, not cross-linked) long-chain silicone molecules

that are mixed together. Silicone (fluid) bleed refers to the diffusion of only small amounts of free (fluid, not cross-linked) silicone molecules through an implant shell; this occurs for all silicone gel–filled implants even when intact, is almost never appreciated on imaging, and is evident on inspection only as a thin slippery lubricantlike coating on the implant surface. When an implant ruptures, the full gel, matrix plus fluid, escapes the implant, sometimes in large amounts. The presence of observable silicone gel outside of an implant almost always indicates implant failure, or rupture. Confusingly, the literature contains references to so-called gel bleed; when those references are referring to silicone gel outside of an implant they are describing implant rupture, and when they are referring to the diffusion of silicone fluid through an implant shell they are describing silicone fluid bleed from an intact

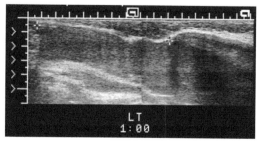

Fig. 22. Extracapsular rupture, large extrusion. The extruded gel (between the *cursors*) is in continuity with gel remaining within the implant and original fibrous capsule.

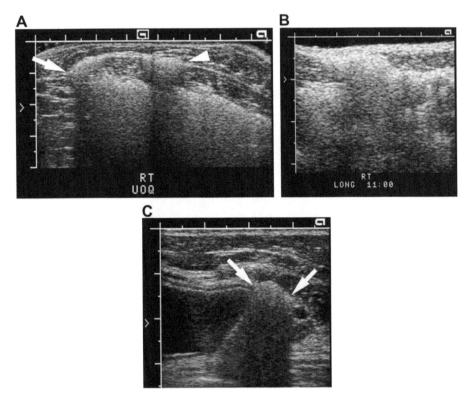

Fig. 23. Silicone granuloma. (*A*, *B*) Multicompartment silicone granuloma. (*A*) Transverse image of silicone granuloma from extracapsular rupture of a submuscular implant with extensive silicone granuloma deep to the pectoralis major, extending around its lateral edge (*arrow*), with some extending into the subglandular space (*arrowhead*) anterior to the muscle. (*B*) Extracapsular rupture of a subglandular implant in another patient, resulting in extension of silicone granuloma into the breast parenchyma and to the dermis of the skin. (*C*) Residual silicone granuloma (*arrows*) contiguous to the edge of an intact subglandular implant. The appearance on this single image could be confused with silicone adenopathy, but the orthogonal image showed that it was irregular in overall shape. The patient had had a prior extracapsular rupture of a silicone gel–containing implant. At the time of explantation, the surgeon did not remove the extracapsular silicone from that rupture.

implant. Thus, silicone fluid bleeds, observable silicone gel that has escaped from an implant, indicates rupture, and the term gel bleed is best not used to avoid ambiguity.[15]

Sonographically, the classic sign of rupture is the wavy-line sign or stepladder sign (**Fig. 18**); however, this is a sign of collapsed rupture. Most ruptured implants that we have seen were not in a state of full collapse (**Table 3**). Therefore, undue reliance on this sign will result in underdiagnosis of rupture with ultrasound. A spectrum of implant shell collapse can be sonographically appreciated. Once the layer of silicone gel is at least a millimeter thick, it may be possible to identify what we have termed the sine sign or drop-away sign. The sine sign is generally seen with thinner shells (**Fig. 19**). The gel on the surface of the implant results in an undulating appearance caused by sagging of the implant shell away from the inner surface of the

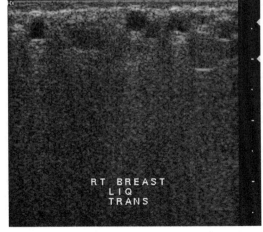

Fig. 24. Direct injection of silicone fluid. Multiple gel cysts within a background of infiltrating silicone granuloma.

fibrous capsule. Initially, only the troughs are visible, because the peaks still touch the inner part of the capsule. With more gel outside of the implant, both the peaks and troughs of the shell can be seen because the peaks are then separated by gel from the capsule as well. With thicker shells and when more gel is outside of the shell, the drop-away sign shows where a sheet of shell has separated from the inner aspect of the fibrous capsule (**Fig. 20**). The appearance is analogous to a false ceiling in a room. Another sonographic sign of rupture is the filled-fold sign (**Fig. 21**).

Rupture can be further delineated as intracapsular when silicone gel is outside of the (outer) implant shell, but confined by the fibrous capsule, and extracapsular, when a rent in the fibrous capsule allows the silicone gel to extend beyond it into soft tissue.

Extracapsular rupture results when the implant is ruptured and there is a breech of the fibrous capsule allowing silicone gel into the surrounding soft tissues. It may present as a focal extrusion of gel into the contiguous soft tissue (**Fig. 22**). If the silicone gel is confined by regrowth of fibrous capsule, a neobiologic capsule, the breech of the fibrous capsule may be manifest only as an apparent bulge in the contour of the implant. A bulge may be caused by herniation of a portion of an intact implant through a defect in the fibrous capsule. Thus, although a focal bulge is usually a manifestation of a form of extracapsular rupture, it is not always so and the implant may be intact.

The trauma that results in a breech of the fibrous capsule (converting an intracapsular to an extracapsular rupture or causing intact implant herniation) may or may not have been sufficient to be noted by the patient.

The entire spectrum of shell collapse, from uncollapsed to fully collapsed, can be seen with intracapsular rupture. Most intracapsular rupture is clinically silent, because the fibrous capsule contains the gel and maintains its form within the breast. With extracapsular rupture, an uncollapsed shell is rare, but the other degrees of shell collapse are often seen. The most common manifestation of extracapsular rupture is silicone granuloma in the soft tissues. Extracapsular rupture is often clinically silent as well.

SOFT TISSUE SILICONE
Silicone Granuloma

Silicone granuloma is the most common manifestation of silicone in the soft tissues from extracapsular implant rupture or silicone fluid injection. The granulomatous reaction results in the silicone being dispersed within the affected tissue as tiny, predominately microscopic cysts. Insonating silicone granuloma results in a characteristic snowstorm artifact. This appearance is likely caused by a complex combination of reverberation and refractions. Silicone granuloma may extend into the breast parenchyma (at times to involve the skin) and along fascial planes for varying distances,

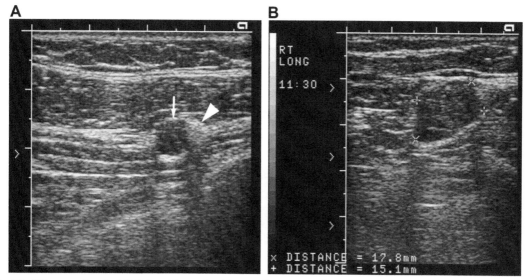

Fig. 25. Silicone gel cysts. (*A*) Gel cyst (*arrow*) with a small amount of contiguous silicone granuloma (*arrowhead*) as the result of extracapsular rupture of a submuscular implant. Note the translation artifact immediately deep to the gel cyst: the anterior margin of pectoralis minor is displaced posteriorly. (*B*) Gel cyst containing echogenic gel. The translation artifact is hard to recognize here because the cyst is not imaged against a long fascial plane parallel to the transducer face.

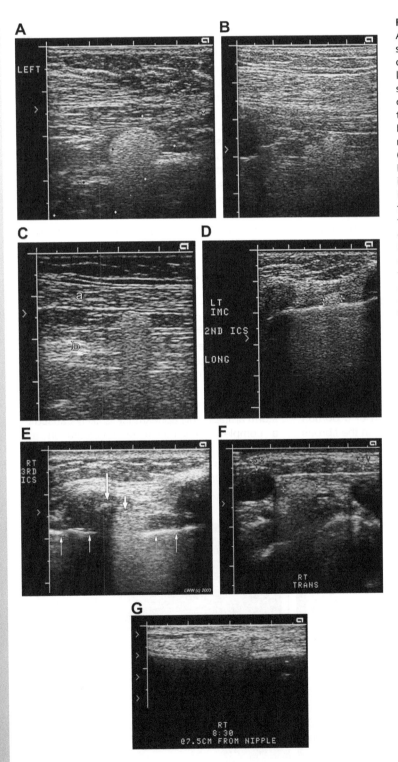

Fig. 26. Silicone adenopathy. (*A*) Axillary level 1. Transverse image showing the typical oval, sharply demarcated appearance. (*B*) Axillary level 2. Longitudinal image showing silicone adenopathy just caudal to the subclavian vessels, the most common location. (*C*) Rotter node between pectoralis major (a) and pectoralis minor (b) imaged transversely. (*D*) Internal mammary chain second intercostal space, longitudinal image. The loss of pleural reflection deep to the node is a typical finding. (*E*) Internal mammary chain third intercostal space, longitudinal image. The node (*small thick arrow*) is just caudal to the costal cartilage, producing a dirty, snowstorm acoustical shadow that prevents visualization of the pleural reflection (*thin arrows*). This shadow is nearly isoechogenic to the lung, but the reverberations caused by the lung move in real time with respiration. Calcification of the costal cartilage (*longer thick arrow*) can also result in obscuration of the pleural bang but it produces a cleaner shadow. (*F*) Supraclavicular node, transverse image. Involvement is most commonly between the internal and external jugular veins, as in this case. (*G*) Intramammary node, transverse image. Within the breast, silicone adenopathy may be difficult to distinguish from silicone granuloma because of a current or prior extracapsular rupture. However, the shape of the affected node is round to oval and the margins are well defined, features that are less common with a granuloma-related current or prior rupture.

occasionally involving the axilla, brachial plexus, and soft tissues of the arm and abdominal wall (**Fig. 23**A, B). When rupture occurs, most silicone granuloma is seen immediately contiguous to the implant, predominately at its radial edge peripherally. Silicone granuloma may be from a prior rupture, and occasionally from silicone fluid bleed, so close correlation of the patient's history and imaging findings is important (see **Fig. 23**C).

In patients with direct silicone fluid injection, which was practiced first in Japan and other parts of the world beginning in the late 1940s, and in the United States mostly from 1963 to the early 1970s (and occasionally even now), injected silicone fluid diffuses widely in the tissues of the breast, including fat, and may be seen within pectoralis and other muscles (**Fig. 24**).

Gel Cysts

Gel cysts are macroscopic collections of silicone gel in the soft tissue that vary from being just perceivable to more than a centimeter in size. They are typically anechoic, and contiguous silicone granuloma is almost always identifiable. If the posterior wall of the cyst is contiguous to a linear fascial plane, the plane may appear to be displaced posteriorly because of the translation artifact (**Fig. 25**).

Silicone Adenopathy

Silicone adenopathy is most frequently seen when a patient has, or has had, polyurethane-coated

---

Box 1
Causes of confusion and potential error

1. Implant contour bulges can result from herniation of normal or ruptured implant through fibrous capsule, or from extrusion of silicone gel from ruptured implant.
2. Echogenic silicone gel can occur as an isolated finding.
3. Subcapsular waterlike fluid is a normal finding with intact textured and polyurethane-coated implants.
4. A standard double-lumen implant with a deflated (outer) saline-containing lumen is functionally equivalent to (and may have the same MR imaging appearance as) an intact, single-lumen, silicone gel–filled implant.
5. Silicone adenopathy should not be confused with silicone granuloma from rupture.
6. Isolated silicone adenopathy in the absence of rupture may occur, as well as silicone adenopathy in the presence of rupture.

---

implants, ruptured or intact. It is believed that the polyurethane promotes the phagocytosis of silicone fluid by macrophages and that the macrophages deposit the silicone within the nodes. Involved nodes can be in any of the lymphatic drainage pathways of the breast and typically are round to oval, well defined, and show the dirty snowstorm acoustical shadowing. Only rarely can the hilum still be identified. These nodes are generally not enlarged; we have seen them as small as 2 to 3 mm (**Fig. 26**). Silicone adenopathy can occasionally occur in the setting of a current (or prior) ruptured silicone gel–filled implant, but

---

Box 2
Imaging pitfalls

1. Redundant or complex folds of an intact implant may simulate a wavy-line (stepladder/linguine) sign of rupture (**Fig. 27**). MR imaging may be necessary for clarification of implant status.
2. The shell pattern of normal, intact, multilumen implants may have a similar appearance to the wavy-line (stepladder/linguine) sign of rupture (**Fig. 28**). History and the mammographic appearance may be helpful, but MR imaging may be necessary.
3. Application of exuberant pressure during sonography can result in a pseudo-sine sign (**Fig. 29**).
4. Textured-surface and polyurethane-coated implants with waterlike fluid outside the implant shell but inside the fibrous capsule can be confused with standard double-lumen implants (**Fig. 30**). The presence of subcapsular waterlike fluid outside an implant should not be confused with silicone gel outside the (outer) shell of a ruptured implant.
5. Misclassification of implant type can also result from exuberant scanning pressure during sonography (**Fig. 31**).
6. Apparent pseudo-debris, which could suggest contamination within a saline-filled implant, or increase in silicone gel echogenicity within a silicone gel–filled implant can be seen when insonating textured-surface implants (**Fig. 32**).
7. A snowstorm sonographic appearance can be seen not only with soft tissue silicone in the parenchyma in the form of silicone granuloma (see **Figs. 23–25**) and silicone adenopathy (see **Fig. 26**) but also can be simulated deep to the shell of textured-surface implants (see **Fig. 7**, **Fig. 9**B, **Fig. 12**C, and **Fig. 32**B). Additionally and rarely, silicone granuloma within the substance of the fibrous capsule can be seen as an isolated finding (**Fig. 33**) in both intact and ruptured implants.

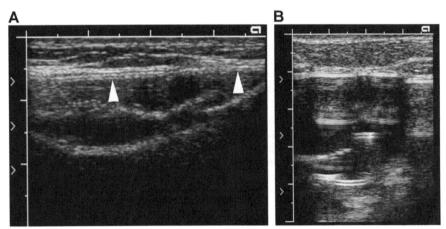

Fig. 27. Pseudo–wavy-line sign: redundant or complex folds simulating the wavy-line sign. (*A*) Intact M Même ME (low profile, single-lumen, silicone gel–filled, polyurethane-coated implant). The shell (*arrowheads*) is apposed to the inner surface of the fibrous capsule. (*B*) Intact Dow Corning P0 14 (low profile, single lumen, silicone gel, smooth shell).

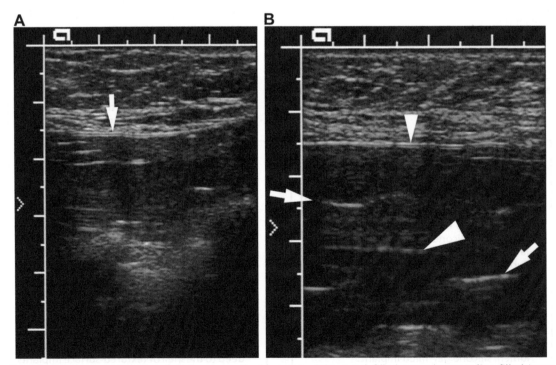

Fig. 28. Pseudo–wavy-line sign: intact, reverse double-lumen (silicon gel–filled outer lumen/saline-filled inner lumen) implants can have an appearance that can be easily confused with a wavy-line sign. (*A*) The only sonographic tip-off suggesting implant integrity is the normal position of the outer shell (*arrow*). (*B*) The outer shell (*small arrowhead*) is in normal position, but the combination of a prominent reverberation (*large arrowhead*) and the incompletely seen anterior and posterior interfaces of the 2 shells (*arrows*) provides for diagnostic challenge.

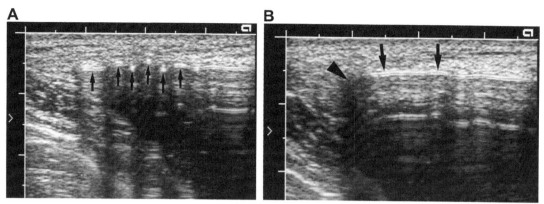

Fig. 29. Pseudo-sine sign. (*A*) Scanning pressure can buckle the anterior surface of the implant, producing a peak-and-trough appearance (*small arrows*). (*B*) Reducing pressure eliminates this effect (*large arrows*). With the pseudo-sine sign, the overlying capsule and soft tissue indents, and remains in contact with the implant shell, peak, and trough, unlike the real sine sign, in which at least the trough and the inner surface of the fibrous capsule are separated by silicone gel. When the shell is no longer parallel to the transducer, the specular reflections from it are lost (*arrowhead* in *B*).

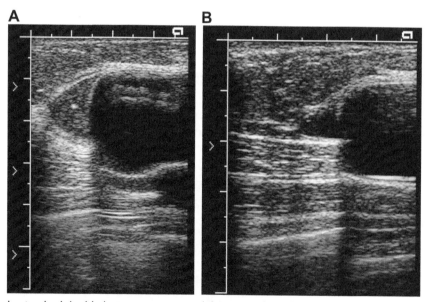

Fig. 30. Pseudo-standard double-lumen appearance. (*A*) Intact polyurethane-coated implant. Note the particles in the waterlike fluid. (*B*) Textured-surface, single-lumen, silicone gel–filled implant. A step-off appearance is noted at the junction of the subcapsular waterlike fluid and the adjacent silicone gel–containing lumen because the latter displays the translation artifact deep to it. History and inspection of the mammogram, looking at the saline-containing lumen, are the easiest ways to make the distinction. A mammogram of these devices will not show an outer lumen, as expected with a standard double-lumen (depicted in **Fig. 14A**). As in this instance, the edge of the inner surface of the fibrous capsule is usually angular when there is subcapsular waterlike fluid and rounded when there is a real outer lumen shell present (see **Fig. 14B**). Recognition of the lack of a translation artifact deep to the subcapsular waterlike fluid helps avoid the pitfall of mistaking the waterlike fluid for silicone gel outside the implant.

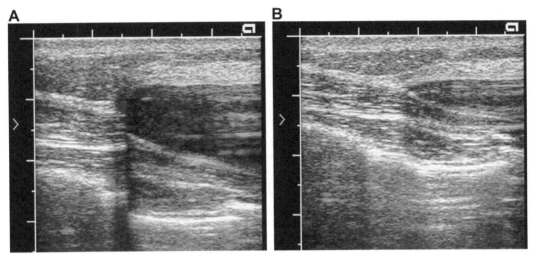

Fig. 31. Effect of scanning pressure on showing the translation artifact: the same single-lumen, silicone gel–filled implant scanned with less (*A*) and more (*B*) pressure. Decreasing the thickness of the silicone gel being insonated diminishes the transit time artifact and can result in a silicone gel–containing implant being confused with a saline-filled implant.

it is uncommon and should not be a criterion of rupture. When a patient has had only 1 set of (intact) implants, silicone adenopathy is only rarely seen unless the implant is polyurethane coated.

Silicone adenopathy is not expected, or seen, in patients who have only had saline-filled implants. Mammography is insensitive in identifying silicone adenopathy.

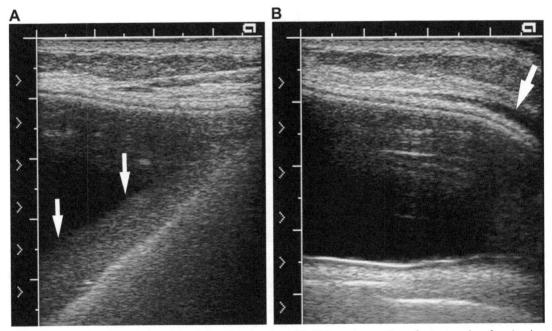

Fig. 32. Simulated debris inside a textured-surface implant. (*A*) Oblique insonation of a textured-surface implant can result in apparent debris posteriorly (*arrows*). (*B*) When the angle of insonation is adjusted to make the posterior border of the implant parallel to the transducer, the artifact within the implant disappears. Some subtle reverberation artifact remains deep to the implant shell. Arrow indicates subcapsular waterlike fluid.

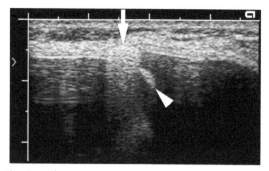

Fig. 33. Silicone granuloma within the substance of the fibrous capsule (*arrow*). The granuloma is seen at the base of a fold (*arrowhead* indicates the tip of the fold). At explantation, the implant was intact and a thickened ridge of fibrous capsule, containing the granuloma, was noted. Granuloma confined to the fibrous capsule of an intact implant is, rare but may be impossible to distinguish from extracapsular silicone granuloma.

CAUSES OF DIAGNOSTIC ERROR AND IMAGING PITFALLS

Several causes of confusion and potential error have been identified (**Box 1**). In addition, imaging pitfalls can also be encountered (**Box 2**).

SUMMARY

Although MR imaging is generally considered more useful than ultrasound to evaluate breast implant–related problems, ultrasound also can detect most implant rupture and is more sensitive than MR imaging in the detection of soft tissue silicone. Rupture detection should be focused mainly on identification of the variable degree of shell collapse that occurs when silicone gel escapes the implant as a whole. Exclusive reliance on only the wavy-line/linguine/stepladder sign results in a loss of sensitivity in detecting implant rupture. Early literature focused on MR imaging and sonographic signs of collapsed rupture and extracapsular rupture, but it is now known that earlier stages of rupture are more common, are evident on MR imaging, and that sonographic signs (the sine sign, drop-away sign, and filled-fold sign) can also detect all stages of collapse of implant rupture. Nevertheless, ultrasound evaluation does have limitations and pitfalls, so correlation with MR imaging may be necessary.

REFERENCES

1. Middleton MS, McNamara MP Jr. Breast implant classification with MR imaging correlation: (CME available on RSNA link). Radiographics 2000;20:E1.

2. FDA. November 2006 PMA approvals. Available at: http://www.fda.gov/MedicalDevices/Productsand MedicalProcedures/DeviceApprovalsandClearances/ PMAApprovals/ucm109790.htm. Accessed November 6, 2010.

3. Agence Française de Sécurité Sanitaire des Produits de Santé. Silicone filled breast implants manufactured by POLY IMPLANT PROSTHESE PIP (01/ 04/2010). Available at: http://www.afssaps.fr/var/ afssaps_site/storage/original/application/ff8f7014c 7016ee7011b6674c7018fb7017dd2835840.pdf. Accessed November 6, 2010.

4. Brem RF, Tempany CM, Zerhouni EA. MR detection of breast implant rupture. J Comput Assist Tomogr 1992;16:157–9.

5. Gorczyca DP, Sinha S, Ahn CY, et al. Silicone breast implants in vivo: MR imaging. Radiology 1992;185: 407–10.

6. Ahn CY, Shaw WW, Narayanan K, et al. Definitive diagnosis of breast implant rupture using magnetic resonance imaging. Plast Reconstr Surg 1993;92: 681–91.

7. Berg WA, Caskey CI, Hamper UM, et al. Diagnosing breast implant rupture with MR imaging, US, and mammography. Radiographics 1993;13:1323–36.

8. DeAngelis GA, de Lange EE, Miller LR, et al. MR imaging of breast implants. Radiographics 1994; 14:783–94.

9. Everson LI, Parantainen H, Detlie T, et al. Diagnosis of breast implant rupture: imaging findings and relative efficacies of imaging techniques. AJR Am J Roentgenol 1994;163:57–60.

10. Soo MS, Kornguth PJ, Walsh R, et al. Complex radial folds versus subtle signs of intracapsular rupture of breast implants: MR findings with surgical correlation. AJR Am J Roentgenol 1996;166:1421–7.

11. Soo MS, Kornguth PJ, Walsh R, et al. Intracapsular implant rupture: MR findings of incomplete shell collapse. J Magn Reson Imaging 1997;7:724–30.

12. Middleton MS. Magnetic resonance evaluation of breast implants and soft-tissue silicone. Top Magn Reson Imaging 1998;9:92–137.

13. Orel SG. MR imaging of the breast. Radiol Clin North Am 2000;38:899–913.

14. Piccoli CW. Imaging of the patient with silicone gel breast implants. Magn Reson Imaging Clin N Am 2001;9:393–408, vii–viii.

15. Middleton MS, McNamara MP. Breast implant imaging. Philadelphia: Lippincott Williams & Wilkins; 2003.

16. Middleton MS, McNamara MP. Breast implants. In: Edelman RR, Hesselink JR, editors. Clinical magnetic resonance imaging, vol. 3. 3rd edition. Philadelphia: Elsevier; 2006. p. 2455–82.

17. Gorczyca DP, Gorczyca SM, Gorczyca KL. The diagnosis of silicone breast implant rupture. Plast Reconstr Surg 2007;120:49S–61S.

18. van Wingerden JJ, van Staden MM. Ultrasound mammography in prosthesis-related breast augmentation complications. Ann Plast Surg 1989;22: 32–5.

19. Levine RA, Collins T. Definitive diagnosis of breast implant rupture by ultrasonography. Plast Reconstr Surg 1990;86:803.

20. van Wingerden JJ, van Staden MM. Ultrasound mammography for the diagnosis of a ruptured breast implant. Plast Reconstr Surg 1990;86:383.

21. Levine RA, Collins TL. Definitive diagnosis of breast implant rupture by ultrasonography. Plast Reconstr Surg 1991;87:1126–8.

22. Peters W, Pugash R. Ultrasound analysis of 150 patients with silicone gel breast implants. Ann Plast Surg 1993;31:7–9.

23. Caskey CI, Berg WA, Anderson ND, et al. Breast implant rupture: diagnosis with US. Radiology 1994;190:819–23.

24. Liston JC, Malata CM, Varma S, et al. The role of ultrasound imaging in the diagnosis of breast implant rupture: a prospective study. Br J Plast Surg 1994;47:477–82.

25. Reynolds HE, Buckwalter KA, Jackson VP, et al. Comparison of mammography, sonography, and magnetic resonance imaging in the detection of silicone-gel breast implant rupture. Ann Plast Surg 1994;33:247–55 [discussion: 256–7].

26. Berg WA, Caskey CI, Hamper UM, et al. Single- and double-lumen silicone breast implant integrity: prospective evaluation of MR and US criteria. Radiology 1995;197:45–52.

27. Venta LA, Salomon CG, Flisak ME, et al. Sonographic signs of breast implant rupture. AJR Am J Roentgenol 1996;166:1413–9.

28. Palmon LU, Foshager MC, Parantainen H, et al. Ruptured or intact: what can linear echoes within silicone breast implants tell us? AJR Am J Roentgenol 1997;168:1595–8.

29. Ikeda DM, Borofsky HB, Herfkens RJ, et al. Silicone breast implant rupture: pitfalls of magnetic resonance imaging and relative efficacies of magnetic resonance, mammography, and ultrasound. Plast Reconstr Surg 1999;104:2054–62.

30. Stavros T, Rapp CL, Parker SH. Sonography of mammary implants. Ultrasound Q 2004;20:217–60.

Lymph Node Sonography

Gary J. Whitman, MD[a],*, Tracy J. Lu[a,b],
Margaret Adejolu, MRCP, FRCR[a,c],
Savitri Krishnamurthy, MD[d], Declan Sheppard, FRCR[e]

KEYWORDS

- Benign lymph nodes • Malignant lymph nodes
- Axillary lymph nodes • Lymph node biopsy

The sonographic appearances of benign (normal and reactive) and malignant (metastatic and lymphomatous) lymph nodes can be explained by an understanding of normal nodal anatomy and nodal pathophysiology. In this article, we review the sonographic features of benign and malignant regional (axillary, infraclavicular, internal mammary, and supraclavicular) lymph nodes. As axillary lymph nodes are those most frequently involved in patients with breast cancer, this review focuses mainly on axillary lymph nodes.

NORMAL NODAL ANATOMY

Lymph nodes are vital immunologic organs distributed widely throughout the body and linked by lymphatic vessels. Lymph nodes are usually small and bean-shaped, and range from a few millimeters to 1 to 2 cm in size. B, T, and other immune cells are stored in and circulate through these lymph nodes, which act as filters for foreign particles. Humans have approximately 500 to 600 lymph nodes, with clusters found in the axillae, groin, neck, chest, and abdomen.[1]

A single lymph node consists of multiple lymphoid lobules surrounded by lymph-filled sinuses and enclosed by a capsule. The smallest lymph nodes may contain only a few lobules whereas large lymph nodes contain many lobules. Lobules within the same lymph node may have different levels of immunologic stimulation and activity; therefore, the lobules will not necessarily have a uniform appearance.[2] There are 3 parts to each lobule: the cortex, the paracortex, and the medulla. The cortex and the paracortex are also sometimes referred to as the superficial cortex and the deep cortex, respectively. The paracortex consists of deep cortical units (DCUs), and each DCU can in turn be anatomically and functionally divided into a central DCU and a surrounding peripheral DCU. Subcompartmentalization of the lobule creates separate areas for T and B cells to interact with their antigen-presenting cells (APCs), and to undergo clonal expansion during times of infection and/or disease.[2]

A single afferent lymphatic vessel delivers a constant stream of lymph to the subcapsular sinus over each lobule. Lymph spreads through the subcapsular sinus at the top of the lobule and flows down the sides of the lobule through the transverse sinuses, and into the medullary sinuses. The medullary sinuses converge at the hilum, and lymph then leaves the lymph node through a single efferent lymphatic vessel.[2]

The space between the lobules of a lymph node is filled with a reticular meshwork made of a delicate, porous, sponge-like tissue. This tissue forms the framework of the lobules and criss-crosses the lumens of the sinuses. The reticular meshwork

[a] Departments of Diagnostic Radiology and Radiation Oncology, The University of Texas MD Anderson Cancer Center, Unit 1350, PO Box 301439, Houston TX 77230-1439, USA
[b] Harvard College, 86 Brattle Street, Cambridge, MA 02138, USA
[c] Department of Radiology, King's College Hospital, Denmark Hill, London SE5 9RS, UK
[d] Department of Pathology, The University of Texas MD Anderson Cancer Center, 1515 Holcombe Boulevard, Houston, TX 77030, USA
[e] Department of Radiology, Portiuncula Hospital, Ballinasloe, Galway, Ireland
* Corresponding author. Departments of Diagnostic Radiology and Radiation Oncology, The University of Texas MD Anderson Cancer Center, Unit 1350, PO Box 301439, Houston TX 77230-1439.
E-mail address: gwhitman@mdanderson.org

Ultrasound Clin 6 (2011) 369–380
doi:10.1016/j.cult.2011.05.005
1556-858X/11/$ – see front matter © 2011 Elsevier Inc. All rights reserved.

inside the lobules, called the lobular reticular mesh-work, is composed of stellate fibroblastic reticular cells (FRCs) whose processes subdivide the lobule into innumerable narrow channels that are occupied by lymphocytes, macrophages, and APCs.[2]

High-resolution ultrasonography allows for clear differentiation of the central echogenic hilum and the peripheral concentric hypoechoic cortex. The hypoechoic cortex, representing the marginal sinus, lymphoid follicles, and paracortex, is thin and has a fusiform shape with smooth edges, while the hyperechoic hilum is attributable to multiple reflective interfaces of blood vessels, fat, and the central sinus (Fig. 1).[3,4]

PATHOPHYSIOLOGY

Lymph arrives via the afferent lymphatics, and filters from the subcapsular/marginal sinus through the cortex and paracortex, via the trabecular sinuses, to the hilum. In inflammatory disease, the diffuse nature of the process is more likely to preserve the nodal shape and the echogenic hilum.[3,5,6] In malignant disease, carcinoma enters the lymph node via the afferent lymphatics, penetrates the capsule, and enters the subcapsular sinus.[6,7] Metastatic disease is arrested in the periphery of the nodes, causing cortical enlargement, which may be eccentric. Consequently, a cortical bulge often precedes generalized cortical enlargement and distortion or destruction of the intranodal architecture, with loss of the hilum. However, microscopic tumor deposits may not cause changes in lymph node morphology, and consequently may be invisible sonographically. In addition, some gross morphologic features seen in malignant nodes may be observed in benign hypertrophic inflammatory nodes.

Sonographic features that have been used to characterize lymph nodes as benign or malignant include size, shape, presence or absence of an echogenic hilum, cortical morphology, echogenicity, nodal border, calcification, cystic change/necrosis, and vascular patterns. There is, however, no one morphologic feature that is specific for malignancy or benignity, although there are combinations of sonographic features (lymph node patterns) that are suggestive of malignancy or benignity, and that may help in determining whether a biopsy should be performed.

Presence of Lymph Nodes

In early reports, the identification of axillary lymph nodes was considered to represent enlargement and therefore metastatic disease.[8–10] With modern high-resolution ultrasonography, lymph nodes are identified in all patients. Women with and without breast cancer have benign axillary lymph nodes.[11,12] Therefore, the mere presence of axillary lymph nodes does not indicate malignancy.

Size

Size cannot be used as the sole criterion in differentiating benign (normal and reactive) from malignant (metastatic or lymphomatous) lymph nodes (Fig. 2).[3,13–17] Microscopic metastatic deposits in axillary lymph nodes, beyond the resolution of existing imaging technology, occur in 9% of patients[11] and therefore it is unlikely that any imaging technique will have a sensitivity greater than 91%. While larger nodes have a higher incidence of malignancy (80% positive predictive value [PPV] if the long axis is >2 cm), reactive nodes can be large and malignant nodes can be small. There is a significant overlap in size between benign (Fig. 3) and malignant lymph nodes, and attempting to differentiate based solely on maximal size is unreliable. There is less overlap using short axis rather than long axis dimensions (90% PPV if short axis is >1 cm).[15,18,19] Using a smaller cutoff value can

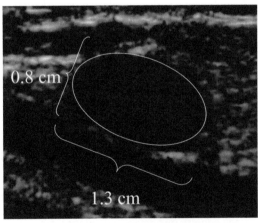

Fig. 2. Small (long axis <2 cm and short axis <1 cm) malignant axillary lymph node.

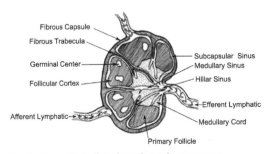

Fig. 1. Normal axillary lymph node anatomy.

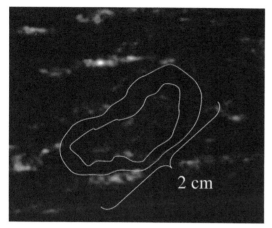

Fig. 3. Large (long axis >2 cm) benign axillary lymph node.

give very high sensitivities but at the expense of a lower specificity.[20]

Shape

Malignant lymph nodes, including nodes involved by lymphoma, tend to be round, whereas normal and reactive nodes tend to be oval or elliptical. The degree of roundness is assessed by using the longest-to-shortest axis ratio (L/S). Reported sensitivities for malignancy using an L/S ratio <2 (ie, more rounded) are approximately 85%, with specificities varying from 61% to 85%.[3,5,21] The reported average cancer content by volume in lymph nodes with an L/S ratio >2.0 was 26%, compared with 59.1% in lymph nodes with an L/S ratio <2.0.[3,5,22,23] Malignant lymph nodes are, however, frequently oval (Fig. 4).

Echogenic Hilum

Previously, the presence or absence of a central echogenic hilum had been proposed as a reliable indicator of benignity or malignancy.[3,4,21,23,24] While the absence of a hilum is very suggestive of malignancy, the presence of a hilum does not

necessarily imply benignity.[3,24,25] The hilum may be absent in 14% of normal lymph nodes,[26] and up to 30% of malignant lymph nodes may retain their hili.[26] As tumor infiltrates the hilum there is loss of the normal echogenicity, resulting in apparent narrowing (hilar compression), hilar displacement (the hilum, rather than lying in the center of the node, lies to one side of the node in at least one plane), and subsequent disappearance of the central hilum (Fig. 5).[5] In some benign lymph nodes, the node is largely replaced by a hyperechoic hilum with no visible cortex demonstrable. The lymph nodes of older patients or patients on chemotherapy may be small and have an isoechoic or a hyperechoic appearance.[27]

Cortical Morphology

The appearances of the hilum and cortex must be interpreted together. Concurrent changes in the shape of the central echogenic hilum and the peripheral concentric hypoechoic cortex may suggest the presence of nodal disease even in the absence of nodal enlargement.[3] The normal cortical rim measures 1 to 2 mm (Fig. 6).[12,13] Neoplastic involvement of the cortex may not affect the cortical echogenicity, but may result in concentric or eccentric cortical widening (Fig. 7).[5,15] Malignant lymph nodes may demonstrate cortical thickening with or without hilar displacement (Figs. 8 and 9). Eccentric cortical hypertrophy measuring greater than 2 mm has been reported

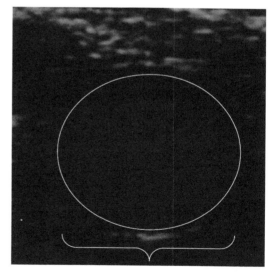

Fig. 5. Malignant axillary lymph node. A rounded (L/S ratio <2), hypoechoic (no visible hilum), 1.5-cm (short axis >1 cm) lymph node. This combination of sonographic features is highly suggestive of malignancy.

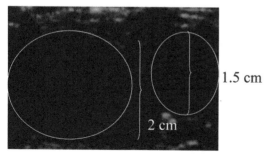

Fig. 4. Rounded and oval malignant axillary lymph nodes.

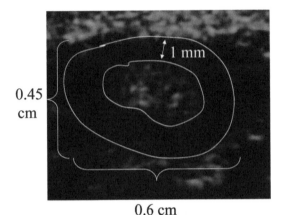

Fig. 6. Benign axillary lymph node. A small oval lymph node (long axis <2 cm, short axis <1 cm) with a thin cortex (<3 mm) and a central hilum (no compression or displacement). This combination of sonographic features is highly suggestive of benignity.

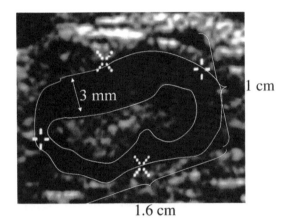

Fig. 8. Malignant axillary lymph node. A small lymph node (long axis <2 cm, short axis >1 cm) with an asymmetrically thickened (>3 mm) cortex with hilar compression (although no hilar displacement). This combination of sonographic features is suggestive of malignancy.

as suggestive of malignancy.[13] It has also been reported that eccentric cortical widening occurs only in malignancy,[3] and that focal doubling of the cortical rim thickness is specific for malignancy. Eccentric cortical widening may be due to focal nodular areas of intranodal metastatic disease.[23] Other studies have used differing cortical thickness cutoff values (3 mm, 4 mm, 5 mm, and 6 mm) with the usual trade-off of decreasing specificity with increasing sensitivity and vice versa. Although a lymph node with a narrow or concentrically wide cortex is generally felt to be benign, there are reports of concentric widening in malignant lymph nodes.[5]

Echogenicity

There have been several reports looking at the internal echo patterns in lymph nodes. Benign nodes are typically reported as being homogeneous, whereas malignant lymph nodes are typically heterogeneous and hypoechoic (**Fig. 10**).[11,19,26,28–31] However, malignant nodes may be homogeneous[17,26,28] and benign lymph nodes may be hypoechoic.[19] Alterations in echogenicity in benign nodes may be due to infection or hemorrhage, and these findings may be mistaken for metastatic disease.[29] Hyperechoic nodes are

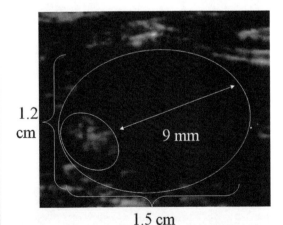

Fig. 7. Malignant axillary lymph node. A small lymph node (long axis <2 cm, short axis >1 cm) with an asymmetrically thickened (>3 mm) cortex with hilar displacement (although no hilar compression). This combination of sonographic features is suggestive of malignancy.

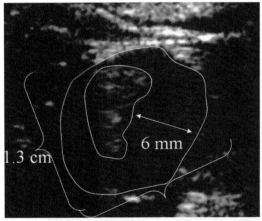

Fig. 9. Malignant axillary lymph node. A small lymph node (long axis <2 cm, short axis >1 cm) with an asymmetrically thickened (>3 mm) cortex with hilar compression and hilar displacement. This combination of sonographic features is suggestive of malignancy.

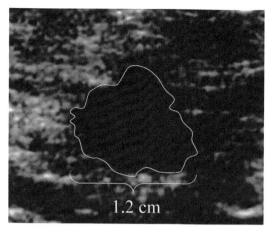

Fig. 10. Malignant axillary lymph node. An ill-defined, lobulated, hypoechoic (with no visible hilum), 1.2-cm (short axis >1 cm), rounded (L/S ratio <2) lymph node. This combination of sonographic features is suggestive of malignancy.

typically believed to be inflammatory,[31] although focal hyperechoic areas can be seen in malignant nodes.[17] Lymphomatous nodes may demonstrate a pseudocystic appearance with hypoechogenicity and posterior enhancement (**Fig. 11**). True cystic change and/or intranodal necrosis is unusual in lymphoma except after treatment. A micronodular pattern has also been reported in lymphoma. Microcalcifications in lymph nodes have been described in the neck in the setting of papillary thyroid cancer. Calcifications in axillary nodes are less commonly reported, but these findings have been reported in treated lymphoma.

Nodal Borders

Benign nodes often have indistinct borders whereas malignant nodes tend to have well-defined borders,[26,28,30,31] due to altered echogenicity in

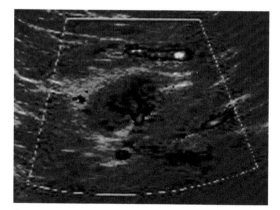

Fig. 11. Lymphomatous lymph node demonstrating hilar and peripheral vascularity.

the replaced node compared with the surrounding tissue. However, with local infiltration, the borders of malignant lymph nodes may become indistinct.[19,23,25] Nodal borders are therefore not reliable predictors of benignity or malignancy.

Vascular Patterns

Small nodes (benign or malignant) may have no demonstrable blood flow because the vessels are small, but flow is demonstrated in 90% of nodes measuring greater than 5 mm. In metastatic lymph nodes, angiogenesis factors may stimulate the growth of new vessels with thin walls, leading to high systolic and diastolic flow and abnormal vascular shunting, resulting in abnormal flow patterns and angioarchitecture.

Normal and reactive lymph nodes may be avascular or have only hilar vascularity. Mixed hilar and peripheral vascularity is associated with lymphoma, whereas pure peripheral vascularity is reportedly more suggestive of metastatic disease.[19,21,32,33] Tumor deposits within a lymph node may compress the intranodal vessels, with resultant increased vascular resistance.[21,32,34,35]

Yang and colleagues[36] evaluated the reliability of unenhanced and echo-enhanced color Doppler ultrasonography in distinguishing benign breast masses and axillary lymph nodes from malignant masses and axillary lymph nodes in patients with known breast cancer. Thirty-two enlarged axillary lymph nodes in 32 patients with invasive cancer underwent power Doppler sonography with and without contrast material. Vascular features and contrast material transit times were recorded. The investigators found that the significant predictors of lymph node malignancy were an increase in peripheral vessel number after contrast material administration and duration of enhancement. Yang and colleagues also found that malignant lymph nodes were enhanced more than the corresponding primary breast cancers, whereas benign lymph nodes were enhanced less than the primary breast tumors.

PATTERNS

No single sonomorphological feature reliably differentiates benign, reactive, or malignant (metastatic or lymphomatous) lymph nodes. Combinations of features either as nodal patterns or as scoring systems better differentiate benign from malignant nodes (**Fig. 12**).[5,19]

Mills and colleagues[37] conducted a retrospective study of 653 consecutive patients presenting with mixed histologic types of invasive breast cancer. The investigators performed 232 ultrasound-guided axillary lymph node biopsies, resulting in

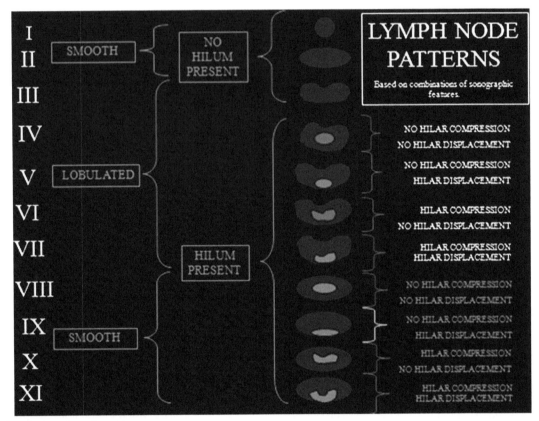

Fig. 12. Lymph node patterns.

a positive diagnosis in 150 cases. The morphologic criteria for metastatic involvement of lymph nodes on ultrasonography were diffuse or focal cortical thickening of more than 2 mm, replacement of the fatty hilum, and abnormal or increased peripheral blood flow. Mills and colleagues found that axillary ultrasound assessment with selected fine-needle aspiration (FNA) or core needle biopsy had a sensitivity of 59%, a specificity of 100%, a PPV of 100%, a negative predictive value (NPV) of 79%, and an accuracy of 84% in the diagnosis of axillary lymph node metastases.

Bedi and colleagues[38] performed high-resolution in vitro sonography on 171 lymph nodes from 19 axillae in 18 patients with unknown axillary nodal status who underwent axillary lymph node dissection for early invasive breast cancer. Each lymph node was classified into 1 of 6 types based on the cortical morphologic features. Type 1 lymph nodes were hyperechoic with no visible cortex; type 2 had a thin (<3 mm) hypoechoic cortex; type 3 had a hypoechoic cortex thicker than 3 mm; type 4 had a generalized lobulated hypoechoic cortex; type 5 had focal, hypoechoic cortical lobulations; and type 6 had a totally hypoechoic lymph node with

no hilum. Types 1 to 4 were considered benign whereas types 5 and 6 were considered metastatic. Interobserver agreement was 77% for classification of nodal morphology (types 1–6) and 88% for characterization of a lymph node as benign or malignant. The NPVs of types 1 to 4 were 100%, 100%, 93%, and 89%, respectively. The PPVs of types 5 and 6 were 29% and 58%, respectively. Sensitivity, specificity, PPV, NPV, and overall accuracy for cortical shape in the prediction of metastatic involvement of axillary lymph nodes were 77%, 80%, 36%, 96%, and 80%, respectively.

Cho and colleagues[39] prospectively evaluated the role of axillary lymph node classification on sonography in 191 patients. The axillary lymph node that had the thickest cortex was prospectively classified on a scale of 1 to 6 according to the cortical thickness and then removed following sonographically guided needle localization and surgical excision. The rates of malignancy, according to the sonographic classification, were as follows: 2% for grade 1 (cortical thickness <1.5 mm), 6% for grade 2 (cortical thickness >1.5 mm and ≤2.5 mm), 40% for grade 3 (cortical thickness >2.5 mm and ≤3.5 mm), 70% for grade 4 (cortical thickness >3.5 mm with an intact fatty hilum), and 90% for grade 5 (cortical thickness >3.5 mm with loss of the fatty hilum). When a cutoff point of a cortical thickness of 2.5 mm was used for determining the presence of malignancy, the sonographic classification showed a sensitivity of 85% (35/41), a specificity of 78% (117/150), an NPV of 95% (117/123), a PPV of 51% (35/68), and an accuracy of 80% (152/191) for the diagnosis of axillary lymph node metastases.

Combining sonographic features such as the presence or absence of a hilum, hilar compression, hilar displacement, smooth or lobulated borders, short axis size, and cortical thickening, it is possible to predict with reasonable accuracy those lymph nodes that are suspicious for malignancy (**Fig. 13**).

LYMPH NODES AFFECTED BY BREAST CANCER

Axillary, infraclavicular, internal mammary, and supraclavicular lymph nodes are located in close proximity to the breast, and these lymph nodes are the most commonly affected nodes in patients with breast cancer. In addition, intramammary nodes may be involved by breast cancer and by lymphoma.

Metastases from Breast Cancer

When cancer metastasizes, nearby lymph nodes are usually affected earlier than distant lymph nodes. Regarding breast cancer, the malignancy metastasizes first to the nearby axillary lymph nodes then to more distant axillary lymph nodes.[40]

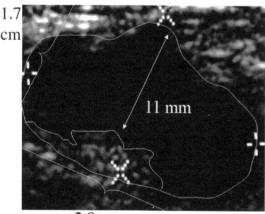

Fig. 13. Malignant axillary lymph node. A large (long axis >2 cm, short axis >1 cm) lymph node with an asymmetrically thickened (>3 mm) cortex with hilar compression and hilar displacement. This combination of sonographic features is highly suggestive of malignancy.

Thus, metastases to lymph nodes are viewed as indicators of tumor progression. Nodal status is also considered a marker of tumor biology, with node-positive tumors having a worse prognosis than node-negative tumors.[40,41] Furthermore, according to studies by Jatoi and colleagues[40] and Nouh and colleagues,[41] there is a correlation between the number of lymph nodes involved and the aggressiveness of the cancer. The total number of lymph nodes involved is more important than the extent to which the disease has spread within the nodes.[42]

As breast cancers increase in size, the likelihood of axillary lymph node involvement increases. In a study of 3747 mastectomy specimens by Nouh and colleagues,[41] 71.6% of T1 (≤2 cm) tumors metastasized to lymph nodes, along with 75.4% of T2 (2–5 cm) tumors, and 85% of T3 (>5 cm) tumors. Multiple tumors were almost twice as likely as single tumors to result in lymph node metastases (24.1% vs 12.4%, respectively).

Tumor grade is a measure of the amount of differentiation in the cancer cells of the tumor, with grade 1 being the most differentiated with a better prognosis, and grade 3 being the least differentiated with a worse prognosis. Node positivity showed a marked increase with an increase in tumor grade, as 49.3% of grade 1 tumors were node positive compared with 76.8% of grade 3 tumors.[41] A surprising finding in the study by Nouh and colleagues[41] was the effect of the laterality of breast cancer on node positivity. Left-sided breast cancer was less prone to cause metastasis to lymph nodes in comparison with right-sided breast cancer. This conclusion may be explained by the more frequent use of the right arm in the predominantly right-handed population.

LYMPHOMA

Lymphoma is the most common type of blood-related malignancy in the United States. Often the first sign of lymphoma (**Fig. 14**) is lymphadenopathy, or swelling of the lymph nodes. The swelling is initially painless and is usually located in the neck, the axillae, or the groin. There are two major types of lymphoma, namely Hodgkin lymphoma and non-Hodgkin lymphoma, and more than 30 subtypes. Hodgkin lymphoma develops from a specific type of abnormal B cell, whereas non-Hodgkin lymphoma may derive from abnormal B or T cells. Risk factors for lymphoma include chronic infection, immunosuppression, hereditary traits, and autoimmune disease. Autoimmune disease constantly stimulates the immune system, and thus can potentially give rise to irregular cloning of autoimmune cells.

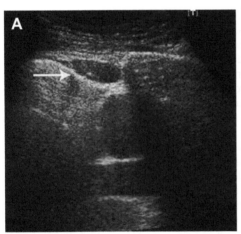
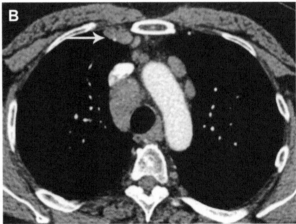

Fig. 14. Lymphomatous involvement of an internal mammary node. (*A*) Ultrasonography shows an oval hypoechoic internal mammary lymph node (*arrow*). (*B*) Computed tomography (CT) shows the suspicious internal mammary lymph node (*arrow*) and additional prevascular and paratracheal lymph nodes.

The diagnosis of lymphoma is often based on lymph node biopsy.[43]

The differentiation of metastatic lymph nodes from lymphomatous nodes (**Fig. 15**) can be difficult. It has been suggested that within the axilla, lymphoma tends to involve all the nodes in a relatively uniform fashion, whereas with carcinoma the lymph node morphology may be different, reflecting differential nodal involvement. With advanced disease, the lymphomatous nodes often become matted together.

SENTINEL LYMPH NODE BIOPSY

The sentinel lymph node is the first lymph node or group of nodes that are expected to be affected by breast cancer metastases. Because the spread of cancer usually follows an orderly progression, a negative sentinel lymph node means that it is unlikely that the cancer has spread to any other, more distant nodes. To assess the sentinel lymph nodes, a sentinel lymph node biopsy is performed. Sentinel lymph node biopsy is advantageous, as it decreases the number of axillary lymph node dissections.[44] Axillary lymph node dissections are more likely to cause postoperative problems such as lymphedema, pain, impaired shoulder mobility, and arm weakness.[45] Furthermore, by identifying the nodes most likely to contain metastases, more attention can be paid to the specific nodes, and micrometastases will have a higher likelihood of being detected.[44] In sentinel lymph node mapping, a radioisotope (usually technetium-99m sulfur colloid), a blue dye (isosulfan blue or methylene blue), or both, are injected before the biopsy is performed. These mapping agents aid in the detection of the sentinel lymph nodes. Studies have shown that the use of both mapping agents yields higher sentinel lymph node identification rates when compared with the use of a single agent.[46] During the procedure, the surgeon uses a gamma probe to detect which nodes have taken up the most radioactive material. These nodes, along with the lymph nodes that have taken up the blue dye, are the sentinel lymph nodes. The pathologist then assesses the sentinel lymph nodes to determine the presence of cancer. Most sentinel lymph nodes are located in the inferior aspect of the axillary region.[45]

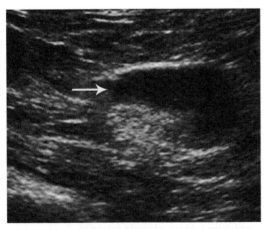

Fig. 15. Sonography demonstrates a 20-mm lymphomatous axillary node with a cortical thickness of 7 mm (*arrow*). The appearance is not specific for lymphoma, and these findings could also represent metastatic disease in a patient with breast cancer.

There are also shortcomings to sentinel lymph node biopsy. There may be false-negative results. Also, cancers may drain by alternative pathways, to the internal mammary or infraclavicular lymph nodes rather than to the axillary lymph nodes. Increasing patient age also affects lymphatic mapping, as sentinel lymph nodes may be more difficult to identify and appear less frequently in older patients.[46]

ULTRASONOGRAPHY WITH CONTRAST AGENTS

Recent reports have noted that sentinel lymph nodes may be identified and localized with contrast-enhanced sonography after the injection of microbubbles. Contrast-enhanced ultrasonography is a developing technique that adds the injection of a contrast agent to traditional sonography.[47] Most studies have used gas-filled microbubbles, and the contrast agent may be administered by intradermal, subareolar, or intravenous injections. Studies targeting sentinel lymph nodes have been performed with intradermal, peritumoral, and subareolar injections.[48–50] The microbubbles have a high degree of echogenicity compared with normal tissue, creating increased contrast in the resulting sonographic images. Lymph node sonography is an area in which the addition of contrast agents may be beneficial, especially regarding identification of sentinel lymph nodes. Contrast-enhanced sonography has the ability to increase the specificity of ultrasound. As ultrasonography with contrast agents advances in the future, its advantages and limitations will be better understood.

PERCUTANEOUS BIOPSY PROCEDURES

In addition to its role in identifying normal and abnormal lymph nodes, sonography plays a major role in guiding biopsies of suspicious lymph nodes. Nearly all biopsies of the regional (axillary, infraclavicular, supraclavicular, and internal mammary) lymph nodes are performed with sonographic guidance. Ultrasound-guided FNA may be performed when adequate cytology support is available. If appropriate cytology support is unavailable, core needle biopsy is suggested. Percutaneous axillary lymph node biopsy determines whether the patient proceeds to sentinel lymph node biopsy or to axillary dissection. Patients with negative ultrasonograms and/or negative ultrasound-guided axillary lymph node biopsies proceed to sentinel lymph node biopsy, while those with metastatic disease documented by percutaneous biopsy will undergo axillary dissection. In addition, patients with proven axillary lymph node involvement will usually be treated with neoadjuvant or adjuvant chemotherapy.

Fine-Needle Aspiration

FNA employs a thin needle (18–25 gauge) to biopsy breast masses and regional lymph nodes. Ultrasonography is used to detect the lymph node in question, and the needle is then inserted into the node and moved in a back-and-forth motion to obtain cellular material under sonographic guidance. Once the cells are extracted, they are stained and evaluated by a cytologist.

In a study by Kuenen-Boumeester and colleagues,[51] ultrasonography combined with ultrasound-guided FNA identified evidence of metastatic disease in 44% (37 of 85) of histologically node-positive patients and in 20% of the patients evaluated in the study. In these cases, cytology identified metastases in the lymph nodes, sparing the patient sentinel lymph node biopsy. In addition, FNA can document extensive metastatic involvement, which may be associated with false-negative sentinel lymph node biopsies.

There is a risk of false-negative axillary lymph node FNAs because the sampling size is small, potentially allowing tumor cells to be missed. Also, FNA may sometimes fail to identify any lymph tissue and instead demonstrate only blood, making the diagnosis inconclusive. In cases where no lymph tissue is obtained, the physician should perform additional passes to retrieve lymphocytes. FNA is particularly useful for sampling deep lymph nodes in the axillary and infraclavicular regions (**Fig. 16**). FNA is a minimally invasive procedure with a low cost and high specificity. When adequate cytology support is available, FNA is a reliable preoperative staging procedure that can eliminate unnecessary sentinel lymph node biopsies.[51]

Core Needle Biopsy

Core needle biopsy removes cores of tissue. Core needle biopsy samples are larger than the samples obtained with FNA. The larger samples allow pathologists to evaluate abnormal cells in the context of the surrounding environment. Ultrasound-guided core needle biopsy is considered to be minimally invasive and safe. In a study by Topal and colleagues[52] of 39 patients who underwent ultrasound-guided axillary lymph node biopsy, the sensitivity and the specificity of ultrasound-guided core needle biopsy of axillary lymph nodes were 90% and 100%, respectively. No significant complications were noted in this study other than pain, which responded to analgesics.

Core needle biopsy is considered a good alternative to FNA when adequate cytology support is lacking. FNA is more dependent on operator expertise than is core needle biopsy. Core needle

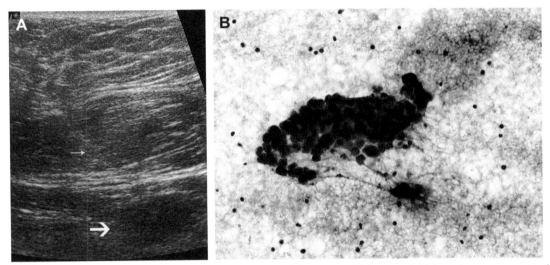

Fig. 16. Metastatic infraclavicular lymph node. A 55-year-old woman with known right breast cancer presented for staging. (*A*) In the right infraclavicular region a deep, suspicious, hypoechoic lymph node was noted. Ultrasound-guided right infraclavicular FNA with a 21-gauge needle (*small arrow*) was used to sample the deep lymph node (*large arrow*). (*B*) Cytology revealed a cluster of tumor cells, representing metastatic adenocarcinoma (Papanicolaou stain, original magnification ×40).

biopsy, like FNA, can be used to document metastatic disease and to avoid sentinel lymph node biopsy. Core needle biopsy has a higher reproducible success rate in comparison with FNA.[45]

SUMMARY

In the future, there will be increased emphasis on sonography of the regional lymph nodes in patients with breast cancer. Gray-scale sonography is an efficient, reliable tool in classifying regional lymph nodes. In addition, ultrasound-guided FNA and ultrasound-guided core needle biopsy are safe, quick, reliable, low-cost procedures that can be used to document metastatic involvement. Contrast-enhanced ultrasonography will likely improve clinicians' ability to classify regional lymph nodes. In addition, contrast-enhanced ultrasonography has the potential to transform sentinel lymph node biopsy into a less invasive procedure.

ACKNOWLEDGMENTS

The authors thank Barbara Almarez Mahinda for assistance in manuscript preparation.

REFERENCES

1. Warwick R, Williams PL. Angiology. In: Warwick R, Williams PL, editors. Gray's anatomy. 35th edition. Philadelphia: WB Saunders; 1973. p. 588–785. Chapter 6.
2. Willard-Mack CL. Normal structure, function, and histology of lymph nodes. Toxicol Pathol 2006;34:409–24.
3. Vassallo P, Wernecke K, Roos N, et al. Differentiation of benign from malignant superficial lymphadenopathy: the role of high-resolution US. Radiology 1992;183:215–20.
4. Rubaltelli L, Proto E, Salmaso R, et al. Sonography of abnormal lymph nodes in vitro: correlation of sonographic and histological findings. Am J Roentgenol 1990;155:1241–4.
5. Vassallo P, Edel G, Roos N, et al. In-vitro high-resolution ultrasonography of benign and malignant nodes: a sonographic-pathological correlation. Invest Radiol 1993;28:698–705.
6. Kendall BE, Arthur JF, Patey DH. Lymphangiography in carcinoma of the breast. A comparison of clinical, radiological, and pathological findings in axillary lymph nodes. Cancer 1963;16:1233–42.
7. Fajardo LF. Lymph nodes and cancer: a review. In: Meyer JL, editor. The lymphatic system and cancer. Frontiers of radiation therapy and oncology, vol. 28. Basel (Switzerland): Karger; 1994. p. 1–10.
8. Bruneton JN, Carmella E, Hery M, et al. Axillary lymph node metastases in breast cancer: preoperative detection with ultrasound. Radiology 1986;158:325–6.
9. De Freitas R Jr, Costa MV, Schneider SV, et al. Accuracy of ultrasound and clinical examination in the diagnosis of axillary lymph node metastases in breast cancer. Eur J Surg Oncol 1991;17:240–4.
10. Mustonen P, Farin P, Kosunen O. Ultrasonographic detection of metastatic axillary lymph nodes in breast cancer. Ann Chir Gynaecol 1990;79:15–8.

11. Bonnema J, van Geel AN, van Ooijen B, et al. Ultrasound-guided aspiration biopsy for detection of non-palpable axillary node metastases in breast cancer patients: new diagnostic method. World J Surg 1997;21:270–4.

12. Yang WT, Ahuja A, Tang A, et al. Ultrasonographic demonstration of normal axillary lymph nodes: a learning curve. J Ultrasound Med 1995;14:821–2.

13. Yang WT, Ahuja A, Tang A, et al. High resolution sonographic detection of axillary lymph node metastases in breast cancer. J Ultrasound Med 1996;16:241–6.

14. Chang DB, Yuan A, Yu CJ, et al. Differentiation of benign and malignant lymph nodes with color Doppler sonography. Am J Roentgenol 1994;162:965–8.

15. Sutton RT, Reading CC, Charboneau JW, et al. US-guided biopsy of neck masses in postoperative management of patients with thyroid cancer. Radiology 1988;168:769–72.

16. March DE, Wechsler RJ, Kurtz AB, et al. CT-Pathologic correlation of axillary lymph nodes in breast cancer. J Comput Assist Tomogr 1991;15:440–4.

17. Maurer J, Willam C, Steinkamp HJ, et al. Keratinization and necrosis: morphological aspects of lymphatic metastases in ultrasound. Invest Radiol 1996;31:545–9.

18. van den Brekel MW, Stel HV, Castelijns JA, et al. Cervical lymph node metastasis: Assessment of radiologic criteria. Radiology 1990;177:379–84.

19. Toriyabe Y, Nishimura T, Kita S, et al. Differentiation between benign and metastatic cervical lymph nodes with ultrasound. Clin Radiol 1997;52:927–32.

20. Van den Brekel MW, Castelijns JA, Stel HV, et al. Occult metastatic neck disease: detection with US and US-guided fine-needle aspiration cytology. Radiology 1991;180:457–61.

21. Na DG, Lim HK, Byun HS, et al. Differential diagnosis of cervical lymphadenopathy: usefulness of color Doppler sonography. Am J Roentgenol 1997;168:1311–6.

22. Tohnosu N, Onoda S, Isono K. Ultrasonographic evaluation of cervical lymph node metastases in esophageal cancer with special reference to the relationship between short to long axis ratio (S/L) and the cancer content. J Clin Ultrasound 1989;17:101–6.

23. Tregnaghi A, De Candia A, Calderone M, et al. Ultrasonographic evaluation of superficial lymph node metastases in melanoma. Eur J Radiol 1996;24:216–21.

24. Yang WT, Metreweli C. Color Doppler flow in normal axillary lymph nodes. Br J Radiol 1998;71:381–3.

25. Evans RM, Ahuja A, Metreweli C. The linear echogenic hilus in cervical lymphadenopathy-a sign of benignity or malignancy? Clin Radiol 1993;47:262–4.

26. Ahuja A, Ying M, King W, et al. A practical approach to ultrasound of cervical lymph nodes. J Laryngol Otol 1997;111:245–56.

27. Spaulding K. Ultrasound imaging of the lymph nodes: normal & abnormal appearance. J Veterinary Radiology & Ultrasound 2008;49:277–81.

28. Ahuja A, Ying M, Yang WT, et al. The use of sonography in differentiating cervical lymphomatous lymph nodes from cervical metastatic lymph nodes. Clin Radiol 1996;51:186–90.

29. Sakai F, Kiyono K, Sone S, et al. Ultrasonic evaluation of cervical metastatic lymphadenopathy. J Ultrasound Med 1988;7:305–10.

30. Noritomi T, Machi J, Feleppa EJ, et al. In vitro investigation of lymph node metastasis of colorectal cancer using ultrasonic spectral parameters. Ultrasound Med Biol 1998;24:235–43.

31. Hildebrandt U, Feifel G. Endosonography in the diagnosis of lymph nodes. Endoscopy 1993;25:243–5.

32. Steinkamp HJ, Maurer J, Cornehl M, et al. Recurrent cervical lymphadenopathy: differential diagnosis with color-duplex sonography. Eur Arch Otorhinolaryngol 1994;251:404–9.

33. Walsh JS, Dixon JM, Chetty U, et al. Colour Doppler studies of axillary node metastases in breast carcinoma. Clin Radiol 1994;49:189–91.

34. Choi MY, Lee JW, Jang KJ. Distinction between benign and malignant causes of cervical, axillary, and inguinal lymphadenopathy: value of Doppler spectral waveform analysis. Am J Roentgenol 1995;165:981–4.

35. Mountford RA, Atkinson P. Doppler ultrasound examination of pathologically enlarged lymph nodes. Br J Radiol 1979;52:464–7.

36. Yang WT, Metreweli C, Lam PK, et al. Benign and malignant breast masses and axillary nodes: evaluation with echo-enhanced color power Doppler US. Radiology 2001;220:795–802.

37. Mills P, Sever A, Weeks J, et al. Axillary ultrasound assessment in primary breast cancer: an audit of 653 cases. Breast J 2010;16:460–3.

38. Bedi DB, Krishnamurthy R, Krishnamurthy S, et al. Cortical morphologic features of axillary lymph nodes as a predictor of metastases in breast cancer: in vitro sonographic study. AJR Am J Roentgenol 2008;191:646–52.

39. Cho N, Moon WK, Han W, et al. Preoperative sonographic classification of axillary lymph nodes in patients with breast cancer: node-to-node correlation with surgical histology and sentinel node biopsy results. AJR Am J Roentgenol 2009;193:1731–7.

40. Jatoi I, Hilsenbeck SG, Clark GM, et al. Significance of axillary lymph node metastasis in primary breast cancer. J Clin Oncol 1999;17:2334–40.

41. Nouh MA, Ismail H, Ali El-Din NH, et al. Lymph node metastasis in breast carcinoma: clinicopathologic correlations in 3747 patients. J Egypt Natl Canc Inst 2004;16:50–6.

42. Lam WW, Yang WT, Chan YL, et al. Detection of axillary lymph node metastases in breast carcinoma by technetium-99m sestamibi breast scintigraphy, ultrasound and conventional mammography. Eur J Nucl Med 1996;23:498–503.

43. Matasar MJ, Zelenetz AD. Overview of lymphoma diagnosis and management. Radiol Clin North Am 2008;46:175–98.

44. Tanis PJ, Boom RP, Koops HS, et al. Frozen section investigation of the sentinel node in malignant melanoma and breast cancer. Ann Surg Oncol 2001;8: 222–6.

45. Abe H, Schmidt RA, Sennett CA, et al. US-guided core needle biopsy of axillary lymph nodes in patients with breast cancer: why and how to do it. Radiographics 2007;27:S91–9.

46. Bonnema J, van de Velde CJH. Sentinel lymph node biopsy in breast cancer. Ann Oncol 2002;13: 1531–7.

47. Wilson SR, Greenbaum LD, Goldberg BB. Contrast-enhanced ultrasound: what is the evidence and what are the obstacles? AJR Am J Roentgenol 2009; 193:55–60.

48. Sever AR, Mills P, Jones SE, et al. Preoperative sentinel node identification with ultrasound using microbubbles in patients with breast cancer. AJR Am J Roentgenol 2011;196:251–6.

49. Yang WT, Goldberg BB. Microbubble contrast-enhanced ultrasound for sentinel lymph node detection: ready for prime time? AJR Am J Roentgenol 2011;196:249–50.

50. Goldberg BB, Merton DA, Liu JB, et al. Contrast-enhanced ultrasound imaging of sentinel lymph nodes after peritumoral administration of Sonazoid in a melanoma tumor animal model. J Ultrasound Med 2011;30:441–53.

51. Kuenen-Boumeester V, Menke-Pluymers M, de Kanter AT, et al. Ultrasound-guided fine needle aspiration cytology of axillary lymph nodes in breast cancer patients. A preoperative staging procedure. Eur J Cancer 2003;39:170–4.

52. Topal U, Punar S, Tasdelen I, et al. Role of ultrasound-guided core needle biopsy of axillary lymph nodes in the initial staging of breast carcinoma. Eur J Radiol 2005;56:382–5.

3-Dimensional Breast Ultrasonography: What Have We Been Missing?

Dennis N. McDonald, MD

KEYWORDS

• Breast • Ultrasonography • 3D • Coronal image

Three-dimensional (3D) or volume ultrasonography, although not new to ultrasound imaging centers, is a relatively new diagnostic tool to most breast imagers. Although volume ultrasonography has gained rapid adoption in cardiac, obstetric, and pelvic imaging, its use in other areas has been limited. Because breast ultrasonography remains predominantly a focused examination, its adoption by breast imagers has been limited to a few progressive imaging centers.

Many consider breast ultrasonography the most difficult ultrasound examination because of the considerable overlap in the appearance of normal fibrocystic change and early pathologic changes that has limited its widespread use. However, with the new generation of multimodality breast imagers, friendlier computer interfaces, improved image resolution, and computer processing capacity, added to the new transducer technology, breast ultrasonography is set to address and overcome many of the limitations of mammography. In addition, breast ultrasonography, specifically volume ultrasonography in the breast, offers a simple, radiation-free, and cost-effective adjunct examination. Volume breast ultrasonography can now offer the kinds of 3D insights previously limited to other modalities, such as magnetic resonance imaging (MRI) and computed tomography (CT). A couple of recent studies have even addressed its use as a successful screening modality in young patients and for those patients with dense breasts.[1,2]

Many believe that 3D breast ultrasonography is poised to offer a new paradigm in breast ultrasound imaging by changing the way imaging is carried out, specifically the way breast ultrasound examinations are acquired, reviewed, and interpreted. In this article, we discuss briefly the physics of volume imaging. We also discuss the principles of volume acquisitions, the advantages and limitations of all volume acquisition techniques, and the suggestions for applications in the busy breast imaging practice.

VOLUME ULTRASONOGRAPHY
Definition

Acquisition of image data from a volume of tissue is known as volume imaging.[3] In ultrasonography, this term is used when discussing 3D and four-dimensional (4D) sonography. Three-dimensional sonography involves acquisition of a volume.

Breast ultrasound has traditionally been a two-dimensional (2D) technique (x-axis and y-axis). The operator acquires a series of 2D static tomographic images and, at times, real-time clips to evaluate a region of interest (ROI). At a minimum, lesions are viewed in 2 orthogonal planes (radial and antiradial). Although other intermediate planes are often imaged when traversing between these 2 planes with conventional 2D imaging techniques, it has been impossible to interrogate breast anatomy in the third orthogonal plane without the acquisition of a volume data set.[4,5]

With advances in computer processing, improved transducer technology, and the need to compete with other volume imaging technologies (ie, CT, MRI), ultrasonography has entered the 3D era. When we say 3D or volume ultrasonography, we are simply referencing the acquisition

Women's Health Center, 625 Steele Lane, Santa Rosa, CA 95403, USA
E-mail address: mcdonadn@sutterhealth.org

Ultrasound Clin 6 (2011) 381–406
doi:10.1016/j.cult.2011.05.003
1556-858X/11/$ – see front matter © 2011 Elsevier Inc. All rights reserved.

and display of spatial anatomy. Similar to the serial acquisition of multiple axial tomographic slices with CT and MRI, multiple 2D slices are acquired with ultrasonography. This acquisition technique and computer reconstruction processing offers the ability to interrogate data in the A, B, and C planes while rotating or manipulating all data on the x-, y-, and z-axis. Four-dimensional volumes on the other hand, combines space and time to give us real-time 3D imaging.[5,6]

The evolution into volume sonography has brought exciting changes to the daily practice of breast ultrasound imaging. Volume ultrasonography has the potential to scan large anatomic areas or volumes producing a data set that can be manipulated to produce multiplanar and 3D images. This data set contains a large number of parallel 2D B-mode images. Furthermore, this data set permits examination of structures in planes that cannot be directly interrogated by the traditional 2D ultrasound beam. In the same manner as with 3D provided with CT and MRI, the lesion or ROI can now be viewed from any projection or plane. Volume review of data sets now offers an entirely new perspective of lesion morphology and regional anatomy, which is refining our ability to better determine tumor extent.[7]

Much of the volume terminology and physics are best understood from the experience and knowledge of MRI and multidetector CT studies. Now with the increasing advancements in ultrasound 3D technologies, the 3D know-how can be applied to diagnostic ultrasonography.

The voxel is the basic element of the volume data set, which provides the benefit of rendering information offering both contrast detail and depth characteristic. A volume then is a 3D array of voxels, just the same way an image is a 2D array of pixels. The combination of the multiple image frames makes up the layers of the voxel. A voxel data set has an appearance similar to a Rubik cube, in which each cube, when used as a unit, allows users to view a single plane in the 3D image volume (**Fig. 1**).[8]

At present, volumetric ultrasound data can be acquired in 2 ways.

1. Manual: free-hand volume sweep

In this method, the operator uses a conventional 2D transducer to sweep through an ROI, simply by moving the probe over the organ and capturing a controlled cine clip of the entire organ or ROI. The overwhelming benefit of this method is that it is cost effective because most ultrasound

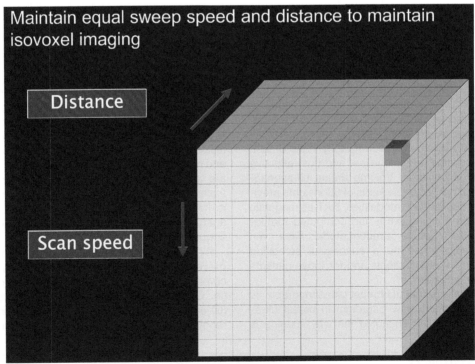

Fig. 1. The voxel is the basic element of the volume data set. A volume is a 3D array of voxels. The goal of any volume acquisition is to have an isotropic voxel data set, that is, a voxel data set that has equal resolution in all 3 planes.

equipments have cine functionality and using the 2D standard probes to acquire clips for volume imaging does not require additional cost in software. The resultant volume data set is a stack of serially acquired 2D image frames. This technique also offers the advantage of not requiring specialized transducers; but because it does not provide spatial reference information, measurements can only be made from the acquisition plane. The advancements in probe position sensor technology may help overcome this limitation.[5,8]

2. Automated: mechanically calibrated transducer acquisition

This technique uses special transducers with internal motors that translate a transducer within the probe housing to scan through a volume of tissue, organ, or ROI, thus acquiring the volume mechanically. Unlike free-hand acquired data, the resultant volumes may be quantified and measurement can be taken in the reconstructed planes of the volume measurements because the acquisition has been standardized. However, these (automated or 4D) transducers tend to be bulky, and their performance may be affected by the unavoidable pressure applied when using these probes. Also, the volume data sets created by these mechanically calibrated transducers can be quite large compared with data sets created with the conventional transducer. Electronic probes could replace these mechanical probes in the future addressing the transducer size issues, but because of the current size of components and the costs of electronic transducers, they are only available for limited applications (**Fig. 2**).[5,8]

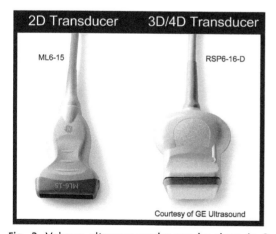

Fig. 2. Volume ultrasonography can be done in 2 ways: (1) manual free-hand volume sweep with a 2D transducer or (2) using mechanical calibrated or electronic 3D/4D transducers.

From any digitally stored volume data set, reconstruction (3D manipulation) is performed on the ultrasound machine console or offline on a picture archiving and communication system (PACS) or independent workstation. With the use of advanced 3D image processing, the information within the stored volume data set can be displayed in any plane regardless of acquisition orientation, which enables the breast imager to virtually rescan a patient by viewing the saved volume in any 2D plane, even different than the original scan plane. You can navigate through the volume in real time using various advanced processing techniques. This navigation enables the practitioner to reorient the ROI to get the best or ideal display. Unlike conventional ultrasonography using 2D still frame capture and review, volume ultrasonography offers real-time cine evaluation of these data as well as 3D volumetric insights previously limited to other modalities.

PRINCIPLES OF VOLUME ACQUISITION

Voxel geometry is affected by several scanning parameters. The goal is to have an isotropic voxel data set, that is, a voxel data set that has equal resolution in all 3 planes so that viewing the data set from any other plane or perspective does not affect the image quality or resolution.

Some of the variables affecting voxel geometry are fixed and not adjustable, whereas others are not and are inherent limitations of current ultrasound technology and 3D reconstruction algorithms. It is beyond the scope of this article to go into the physics of volume acquisition; however, it is necessary to point out certain fundamental principles for acquiring an adequate volume data set for 3D interrogation.

1. The 2D image should be optimized first because the resulting volume data set is compiled from a series of parallel 2D slices or images that represent the volume of tissue scanned. The quality of the 3D image is directly dependent on the quality of the 2D building blocks.
2. When possible, the volume sweep should cover the entire lesion or ROI in a single sweep. Sweeping beyond the lesion at each end ensures that the borders of the lesion have been covered.
3. It is important to maintain a high frame rate when performing a manual volume sweep because more frames firing during the volume cine sweep ensures more data when compiling this sweep into a volumetric data set. Average frame rate for manual volume sweeps is

approximately 30 to 40 Hz. When using the 4D transducers, acquisition parameters must be set to the highest quality settings.

4. In free-hand sweeps scan techniques, aside from higher frame rates, scan techniques such as sweep speed and sweep distance are manually maintained for even slice spacing and global evaluation. The goal is to acquire a volume sweep so that the voxels of data are as nearly isotropic as possible. You want to achieve similar lateral and elevation (in the slice thickness direction) resolution. Using simple settings (30- to 40-Hz frame rate, sweep speed of approximately 1 cm/s, and the greatest distance covered of 6–15 cm), this will result in data that have near-isotropic image quality in all orthogonal planes.

5. Matrix transducers (1.5-dimensional array) can dynamically focus in the elevation plane and produce a thinner ultrasound beam that varies less with depth than the conventional ultrasound transducer. We find them ideal for volume acquisitions in the breast.[3] (Refer to the respective vendor for specific volumetric scanning technique parameters because these parameters vary slightly between vendors [**Figs. 3–5**].)[5,9]

IMAGE OPTIMIZATION

Like any ultrasound examination, volume ultrasonography requires a sonographer who understands the limitations of sonography and the physics of ultrasound to perform a quality study. Image optimization can be a whole article in itself but remains the cornerstone to quality volume ultrasonography. Experience shows that frequently the 2D image has not been optimized for lesion detection and characterization. These parameters change with various situations. Increased knowledge of the different ultrasound scanner settings and their appropriate use improve the quality of the image and, subsequently, the quality of the 3D examination. The pathology must be properly displayed using proper basic imaging techniques. In addition, the number of focal zones should be adjusted to focus the anatomy from the skin to the pectoralis muscle if possible. Harmonics and spatial compound imaging help with contrast resolution and edge definition of pathology (**Fig. 6**).[10]

IMAGE PROCESSING

The processing phase includes enhancing images, segmentation of regions of interest, fusing multimodality images and rendering them in novel ways.

—*Richard Robb, PhD*

The same 3D processing can be performed on the scanner, on the ultrasound machine console, or on a separate 3D workstation (PACS or advanced application 3D workstation). The option you choose often depends on department budgetary allowances and division of workflow. We have independent workstations in my institute, which was a decision based on our workflow dynamics; with the examination time continually being shortened, the sonographer no longer has the luxury of

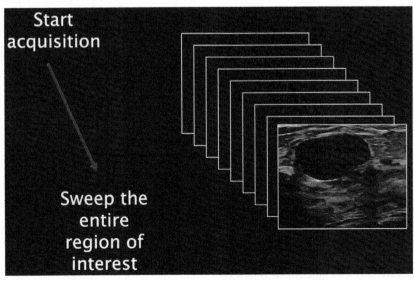

Fig. 3. A volume acquisition using a manual or free-hand volume sweep requires the operator to maintain a constant scan speed while moving the transducer over the ROI.

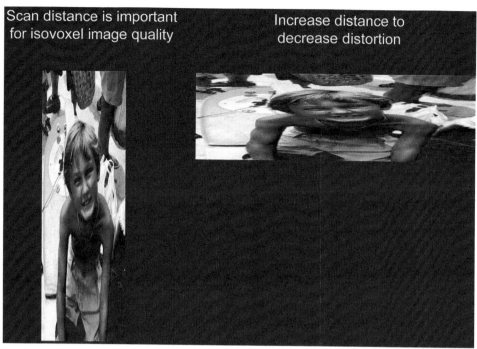

Fig. 4. Voxel geometry is affected by several scanning parameters. Scan distance and scan speed are 2 of these parameters that can affect image quality. It is important to acquire the volume data set with a constant scan speed, but scan distance is also important for isovoxel image quality.

"in room" 3D manipulations. Although, it is important to point out that, because many of these manipulation processes become automated or routine, the time required for reconstruction is

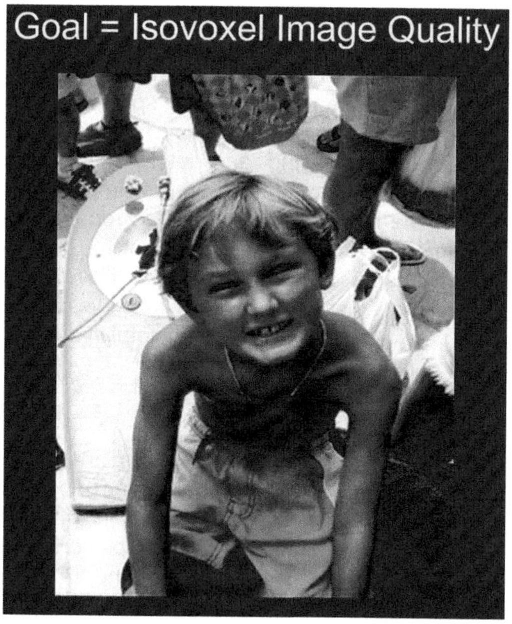

Fig. 5. The goal of any volume acquisition is to have an isotropic voxel data set, that is, a voxel data set that has equal resolution in all 3 planes.

nominal. In addition, there are several factors to consider (**Box 1**).

IMAGE DISPLAY

For many years radiologist have used their 2D examinations to extrapolate and triangulate in their minds a mental 3D reconstruction by going back and forth between the various images. At present, all this has changed; now it is possible to view the coronal plane or any plane that best demonstrates the pathology. For several years other cross-sectional imaging studies (CT and MRI) have had the advantage of 3D display options, such as tomographic sections, multiplanar reformation (MPR), curved coronal reconstruction, and so forth. Three-dimensional ultrasonography once considered by many to be a gimmick, now has these options and is poised to become the standard of care in breast ultrasound imaging.[5]

In 3D imaging it's all about the displays. Three-dimensional display features continue to evolve to better meet the diverse needs of the radiologists and specialists who use them for diagnosis and treatment planning, and, although the 3D era of ultrasonography is in its early stage, there are several display options available to the breast imager. Some of the display options have apparent value in delineating breast anatomy and

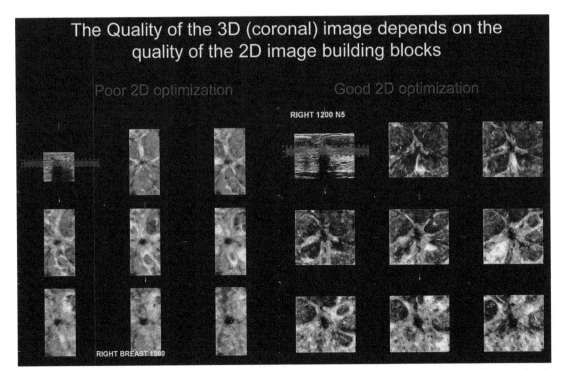

Fig. 6. One of the fundamental principles for acquiring an adequate volume data set is to initially optimize the 2D image because the resultant volume is a series of parallel 2D images that represent the volume of tissue scanned.

pathologic findings, whereas others seem best suited for applications in other anatomic regions (ie, obstetrics, gynecology, cardiology, orthopedics, and so forth).

A 3D sonographic volume contains all the sonographic ROI information within it. Once you have

---

Box 1
Factors in 3D image processing

Machine console

Not all vendors offer the full functionality of an independent or a PACS workstation. Not all vendors have both 3D from a manual sweep and a 3D/4D probe solution.

PACS workstation

As mentioned previously, not all PACS vendors offer full or independent 3D functionality or cine sweep/loops review. Depending on the workstation and the vendor, the ease of use and functions vary. However, shifting the data sets to an independent workstation minimizes disruption of the schedule and allows for dedicated 3D technologists (super users) or even full 3D laboratories workflow solutions.

---

the volume, you now need to use the various reconstruction and rendering algorithms to maximize the extraction of information from any volume data sets. There are many ways to render the volume data sets, and many of the current reconstruction and display options are shared by the various ultrasound vendors, whereas other more advanced options remain vendor specific. Breast imagers find that certain display functions work best for their reading and interpretive styles. Some of the display options are as simple as the push of the button, whereas others require delicate interactive data manipulation to get the desired image. Although it is not possible to discuss every display option available, we discuss those that we have found most helpful in a typical breast center.

1. Multiplanar display

In this approach, the acquisition plane is displayed along with 2 planes that are generated from the data set. The 3 planes are always orthogonal to each other. The A plane shows the original acquisition image, the B plane is orthogonal to A (ie, antiradial plane if A is radial) and C is the coronal plane that is orthogonal to A and B. The operator can navigate through the volume using a single point of reference in all 3 planes viewing its relative location as the planes move (**Fig. 7**).[5–7]

2. Multislice display (tomographic ultrasound imaging)

In this variant of the multiplanar display, the software takes the acquired volume and produces a series of parallel slices. By manipulating interactive controls, the operator can adjust the number of slices, organ or ROI display, thickness or interslice distance depending on vendor options. Images are similar to those typically displayed in CT and MRI. It is possible to slice and document the lesion in all 3 planes (**Fig. 8**).[5–7]

3. Shaded surface-rendered display

Shaded surface-rendered display represents a 3D display of the volume data using gray-scale or color-shading techniques to give an illusion of depth. The fidelity of the resultant image depends on the differences in echogenicity to the adjacent tissues, so when there is fluid within or surrounding the lesion, this can

act as a negative contrast medium permitting better visualization of the lesion margins. It is possible only when an interface surrounded by fluid exists (**Fig. 9**).[5–7]

4. 3D Angio map (3D Doppler display)

This display option goes by various names depending on the vendor. This 3D mode makes the gray-scale data transparent and displays the power or color Doppler data within the volume. This mode offers the basis for a detailed study of the 3D vascular supply of the lesion and the surrounding breast tissue. This studying is more difficult than displaying organ vascularity because tumor angiogenesis involves abnormal vessels that are more easily compressed during the acquisition when too much pressure is applied.[5,6]

5. Interactive volume cube

Interactive volume cube is a 3D representation of the complete volume data set. In both the hand-held and automated acquisitions, minor adjustments to size may need to be made for

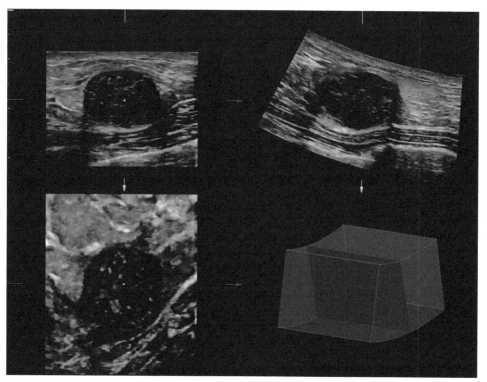

Fig. 7. Multiplanar display. In this display, the acquisition plane is displayed along with 2 planes that are generated from the data set. The 3 planes are always orthogonal to each other. In this example, the A plane (*upper left*) shows the original acquisition image, the B plane (*upper right*) is orthogonal to A (ie, antiradial plane if A is radial), and C plane (*lower left*) is the coronal plane that is orthogonal to A and B (*arrows*).

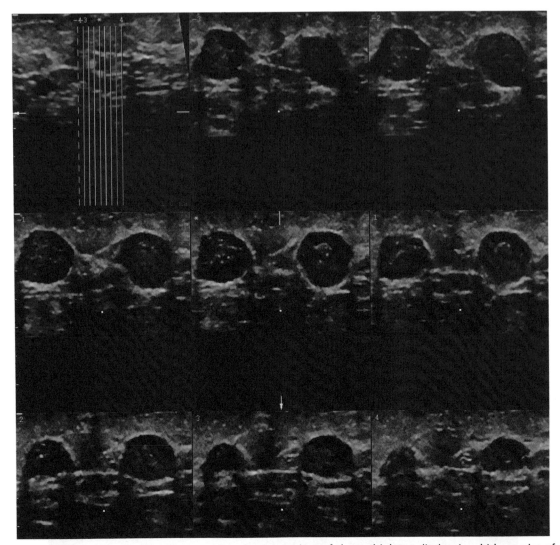

Fig. 8. Multislice tomographic ultrasound imaging is a variant of the multiplanar display, in which a series of parallel images are generated in selected planes. Images are similar to those typically displayed in CT and MRI studies (*arrows*).

isotropic or isovoxel approximation. The user then can interactively view the serial data from each plane or can alter the cube to view from any perspective.[5,7]

Rendering parameters can be varied to visualize different aspects of the acquired volume. Rotation of the volume often is necessary to permit optimal demonstration of pathology. This display offers new ways of visualizing complex anatomy in a 3D image, which were previously difficult to appreciate. Cine loops of the display planes can be re-created which can be very informative for the referring physicians (**Fig. 10**).

6. 3D navigation (virtual rescan)

This is a term given to the most interactive volume manipulation tool. It allows real-time, or on-the-fly manipulation of a single reference point within the volume data set (volume cube). Experienced users find this the fastest way to view and sort out complex anatomic relationships (ie, tumor extension) (**Fig. 11**).[5]

For years we have relied on MPR and tomographic displays when reading CT and MRI examinations. Now there are several tools to efficiently navigate these large data sets with a full spectrum of planar and volumetric display

A   B

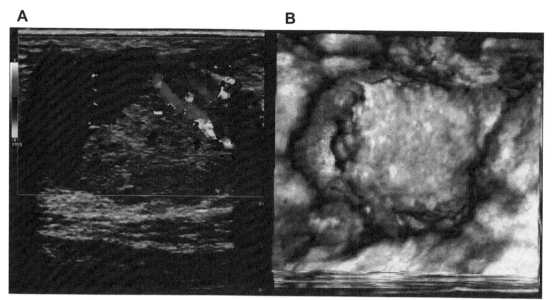

Fig. 9. (*A*) Acquisition and (*B*) shaded surface-rendered display represents a 3D display of the volume data using gray-scale or color-shading techniques to give an illusion of depth. It is possible when an interface surrounded by fluid exits.

techniques that allow use of routine hanging protocols or essentially real-time interactivity and volume exploration of lesion structure, growth patterns, and blood supply.

3D ANATOMIC CORRELATION

Any discussion of 3D breast ultrasonography starts with review of the pertinent anatomy and the correlation of histopathology with the

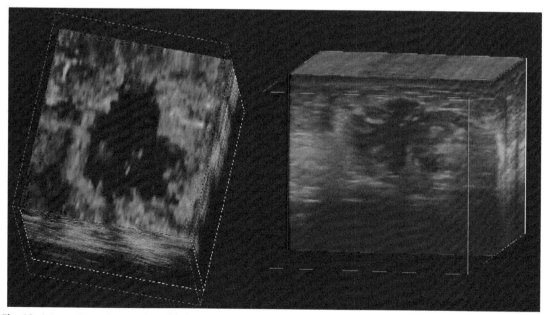

Fig. 10. Interactive volume cube. This is a 3D representation of the complete volume data set. The user can interactively view the data from each plane or can alter the cube to view the lesion from any perspective. Rendering parameters can be varied to visualize different aspects of the acquired volume. This display offers new ways of visualizing complex anatomy in a 3D image.

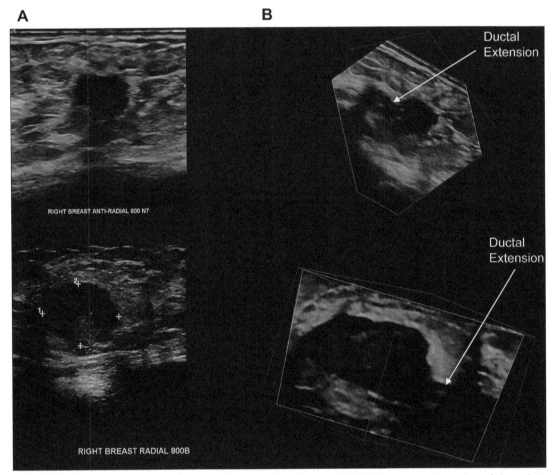

A

B

RIGHT BREAST ANTI-RADIAL 800 N7

RIGHT BREAST RADIAL 800B

Ductal Extension

Ductal Extension

Fig. 11. (*A*) Acquisition image and (*B*) 3D navigation (virtual rescan). This is the most interactive of the volume display options because it allows real-time or on-the-fly manipulation of a single reference point within the volume data set.

sonographic appearance of benign and malignant abnormalities. "The breast is a 3 dimensional structure and the ultrasound appearance is inherently based on 3D-thinking about normal anatomy as well as its deformation, called pathology." (L. Tabar, personal communication, 2010).

The breast ultrasound image varies depending on the relative distribution of the various ductal and parenchymal components. Understanding the basic structural elements and knowing the capabilities and limitations of ultrasonography help in recognizing the normal condition and detecting abnormalities with a greater degree of certainty. It is now possible to identify anatomic zones within the breast, the various tissue types, and several orders of mammary ducts and often the functional unit of the breast, the terminal ductal lobular unit (TDLU).

Dr Tabar and a few pathologists in the United States such as Lee Tucker have given us valuable insights into 3D ultrasonography through thick section (3D) histology and with the use of large-section histology. Thick section pathology, as the name implies, has depth. Unlike traditional histology, large-section histology slices the mastectomy or excisional biopsy specimens in the coronal plane. So why is this important? In large-section histology there is continuity without individual sections separated by several centimeters. Tumor extent, margin analysis, and multifocality are all best demonstrated by this technique (**Fig. 12**).

In the mature female breast, the mammary zone, which contains the glandular elements, lies between the superficial and deep mammary fascia. Breast fat is found beneath the skin, found beneath the glandular tissue, and fills the spaces between the lobes. The adult female breast is composed of 15 to 20 lobes that contain the functional epithelial elements of the breast. The overlapping lobes are arranged generally radially

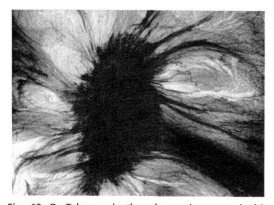

Fig. 12. Dr Tabar and others have given us valuable insights into 3D breast ultrasonography through thick-section (3D) histology. Unlike traditional histology, thick-section histology has depth that allows us insights into the coronal plane. (*Courtesy of* Dr Laszlo Tabar, Falun, Sweden.)

around the nipple. Each lobe contains numerous lobules, which are drained by small branching ducts that unite to form a main lactiferous duct with an opening in the nipple. The lobule is called more specifically the TDLU. The TDLU is composed of multiple ductules or acini, the intralobular terminal ducts and the extralobular terminal duct. For simplicity's sake, we have diagrammed the TDLU in the shape of a badminton racket. There are anterior (most numerous), posterior, and terminal TDLUs. The mammary ducts are oriented in the parallel or coronal plane, and the lobules (extralobular terminal ducts and TDLUs) are oriented in the nonparallel direction with conventional breast ultrasonography (**Figs. 13** and **14**).[7,11,12]

Most benign and malignant breast pathologic conditions arise within the TDLU. Generally the TDLU is only visible in a background of echogenic fibrous tissue. As a rule, the TDLUs that lie anterior to the main lobar ducts tend to have longer extralobular terminal ducts than those located posteriorly, which is probably at least partially responsible for many small cancers having

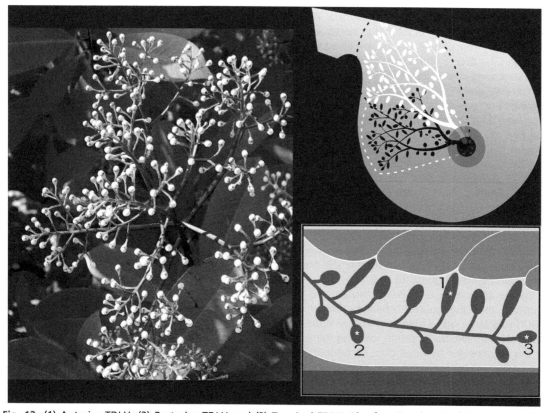

Fig. 13. (1) Anterior TDLU, (2) Posterior TDLU and (3) Terminal TDLU. The functional unit of the breast is the TDLU, which consists of the intralobular and extralobular portions of the terminal duct and the lobule. The lobule is composed of the intralobular terminal duct, ductules (acini), and intralobular stromal fibrous tissue. The lobar ducts drain to the nipple in a generally radial fashion that is similar to the arrangement of the spokes of a wheel. (*Courtesy of* Dr Laszlo Tabar, Falun, Sweden and Tom Stavros, Santa Rosa, CA.)

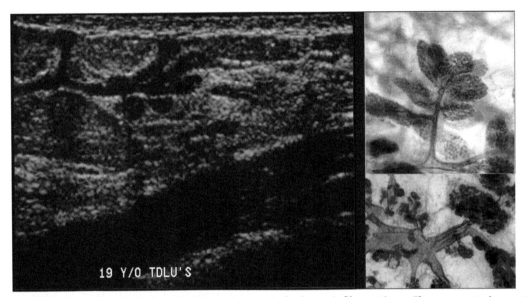

Fig. 14. Generally the TDLU is only visible in a background of echogenic fibrous tissue. There are anterior, posterior, and terminal TDLUs. The mammary ducts are oriented in the parallel or coronal plane, and the lobules (extralobular terminal ducts and TDLUs) are oriented in the nonparallel direction with conventional ultrasonography. (*Courtesy of* Dr Laszlo Tabar, Falun, Sweden and Tom Stavros, Santa Rosa, CA.)

a greater anteroposterior dimension than transverse dimension (taller than wide). Normal TDLUs are usually 1 to 2 mm in diameter; however, the size can vary from patient to patient, with age, location, and the phase of the menstrual cycle. Most breast cancers arise in the TDLU (90%). The breast cancer enlarges and distorts the lobules from which it arises and the ducts through which it spreads. Now how does this influence which plane to image the breast? Tabar has postulated that coronal images that have a thickness less than or equal to the thickness of the normal TDLU may be the optimal plane for breast ultrasound screening, that is, the best plane to demonstrate the earliest change in TDLU morphology. Recognizing these changes at earlier stages and with appropriate treatment improves prognosis (**Fig. 15**).

U-systems/Siemens have incorporated the reconstructed coronal plane into their whole breast ultrasound systems (**Figs. 16** and **17**).

Lander and colleagues[2] have diagrammed this showing that the earliest changes cause the TDLU to enlarge with widening primarily in the extralobular terminal duct portion, causing the waist of the extralobular terminal duct to be lost. The importance of this is that cancers are seen on 4 to 6 coronal images, whereas Aberrations in the Normal Development and Involution of the breast (ANDI) TDLUs are seen on only 1 or 2 images (**Figs. 18** and **19**).[2]

Breast cancer is heterogeneous, that is to say, it varies from one nodule to another and even within an individual nodule. Some breast cancers are

circumscribed with features that overlap with benign lesions. Spiculated breast cancers are at the other end of the spectra. Cancers are known to incite angiogenesis, lymphangiogenesis, and neoduct genesis.

Some tumors incite a desmoplastic response, whereas faster-growing lesions often incite an inflammatory response (lymphocytes, plasma cells, or both). Dr Giorgio Rizzatto found, when researching the biomechanics of breast tissues and cancer, pathology references that document that abnormal paracrine signaling results in large numbers of myofibroblast conversions that secret collagen and fibronectin, which stiffen the tumors (G. Rizzatto, personal communication, 2009). Macrophages contract and help stiffen lesions even further. These metabolic byproducts, enzymes, proteins, and other chemical factors result in desmoplasia, which results in retraction, distortion, and a variety of other changes that alter the surrounding tissues.[11,13–19]

From an imaging perspective, what we visualize is a combination of tumor expansion and infiltration and host response. Like other malignancies, breast cancer often extends in the path of least resistance in the mammary zone, that is, the coronal plane, because of the barrier effect of the anterior and posterior mammary fascia.

CORONAL PLANE

The coronal ultrasound plane is not available using conventional 2D ultrasound imaging because it is

A   B

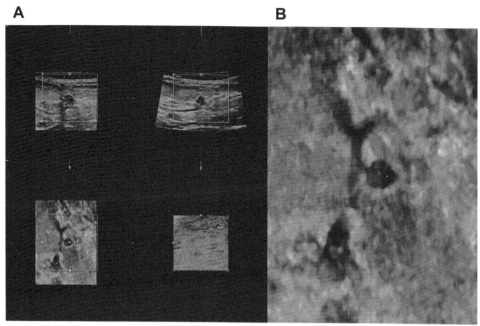

Fig. 15. (*A*) MPR and (*B*) coronal reconstruction. Mammography showed a small nodular asymmetry; however, when viewing this 3D data set in the coronal plane, it is possible to show that this represents a peripheral papilloma arising in a TDLU (*arrows*).

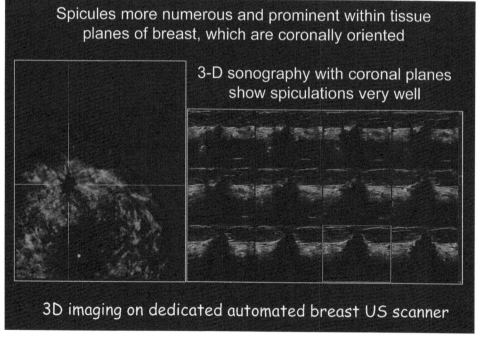

Fig. 16. Another example of multislice display capability with a biopsy-proved malignancy. Not only is the lesion better represented on the coronal view with its relationship to the surrounding architecture but also the multislice display easily shows the best point to make an accurate measurement. (*Courtesy of* U-systems, Sunnyvale, CA and M. Lander, Palm Spring, CA.)

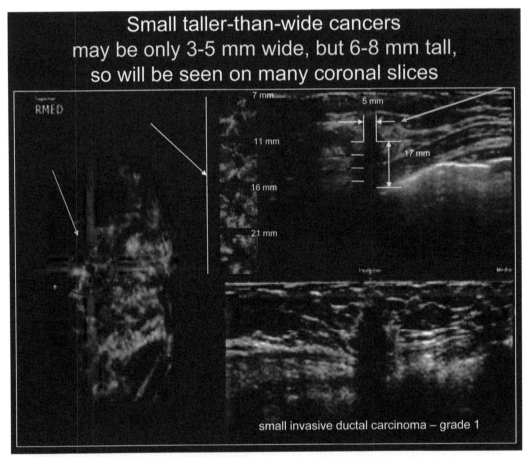

Fig. 17. U-systems SomoSynthesis (Sunnyvale, CA) combines tissue signals from multiple adjacent scan planes using voxel synthesis. Here is an example of a small invasive ductal carcinoma that is only 5 mm in size. Traditional 2D hand-held scanning would be limited to the information visible only in 3% of the 2D slices. But because of its associated acoustic shadow and the 3D information provided through voxel synthesis, the coronal view demonstrates the lesion in 30% of the displayed slices (*arrows*). (*Courtesy of* U-systems, Sunnyvale, CA and M. Lander, Palm Spring, CA.)

the view parallel to the probe face and perpendicular to the ultrasound beam. To fully understand the importance of the coronal plane in breast imaging, one needs to look at breast anatomy and the unique features that make imaging in the coronal plane so helpful to the breast imager.

There is no way of predicting the desired angle for viewing pathologic abnormalities; however, we have found the coronal plane extremely valuable and that it is easily obtained and displayed.[4] As discussed earlier, the coronal plane offers an additional perceptual opportunity to detect early breast cancer by identifying serial images of the altered TDLU or the architectural distortion seen with invasive lesions. This plane allows us to better understand and visualize the early lesion surface changes and the associated changes in the surrounding mammary and supporting tissues.

The coronal plane most accurately displays tumor growth patterns allowing the reviewer to visualized microlobulations, angular margins, and spiculations. Several investigators have noted that breast cancers typically demonstrate a pattern of retraction and compression (architectural distortion), which is readily demonstrated in the coronal plane. Spiculation and disrupted Cooper ligaments and changes in the shape and disruption of the superficial fascia can be seen with 2D images; however, these findings are more impressive in the coronal plane. Even in small cancers (<1 cm), the retraction pattern is visible in the coronal plane (**Fig. 20**).[8,9,13–18,20]

Waterman and colleagues[8] found the retraction phenomenon in the coronal plane of 3D ultrasonography to be a significant and independent factor for lesion characterization. We have found

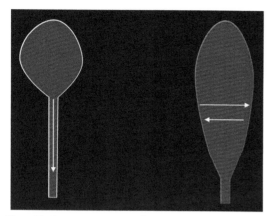

Fig. 18. Breast cancer enlarges and distorts the lobules from which it arises and the ducts through which it spreads. The earliest changes cause the TDLU to enlarge with widening primarily in the extralobular terminal duct portion, causing the waist of the extralobular terminal duct to be lost. (*Courtesy of* M. Lander, Palm Spring, CA and Dr Laszlo Tabar, Falun, Sweden.)

that most breast cancers demonstrate this retraction phenomenon, however, not all, and we are currently reviewing our last 700 breast cancers with 3D data sets to see exactly what morphologic characteristics, biomarkers, and histologic features are seen with these changes. We hope that the combination of a negative coronal plane and elastography examination may eventually eliminate the need for 6-month short-term follow-up ultrasonography in some probably benign breast lesions and

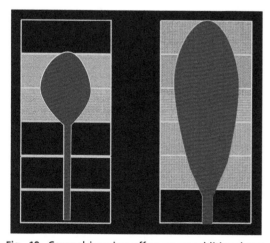

Fig. 19. Coronal imaging offers us an additional perceptional opportunity to detect early breast cancer either by identifying serial images of the altered TDLU or the architectural distortion seen with invasive lesions. Cancers are seen on 4 to 6 coronal images and Aberrations in the Normal Development and Involution (ANDI) TDLU on only 1 or 2 images. (*Courtesy of* M. Lander, Palm Spring, CA and Dr Laszlo Tabar, Falun, Sweden.)

that the routine use of the coronal plane may help us refine the classification of Breast Imaging–Reporting and Data System (BI-RADS) 4 lesions (**Figs. 21** and **22**).

Differential diagnosis of irregular or spiculated masses

- Carcinoma
- Surgical scar
- Fat necrosis
- Radial scar
- Abscesses
- Granular cell tumor.

Because of the heterogeneous nature of breast cancer, you can observe a spectrum of findings from spiculations to architectural distortion, and it may not be possible to differentiate between the two on an individual lesion basis (**Fig. 23**).

We have found that pathologic areas of architectural distortion on mammography are readily identified in the coronal plane on ultrasonography and that mammographic distortion without ultrasound correlate is almost universally because of superimposition of tissue that typically effaces with additional mammographic evaluation. Our current protocol takes patients directly from mammography to ultrasonography for architectural distortion. If an abnormality is noted on coronal ultrasound imaging, the patient is scheduled for an ultrasound biopsy.

The coronal plane can also confirm benign causes to frequently encountered masses and may lend additional information on intraductal pathology for intervention and surgical planning. The coronal plane often provides a more understandable representation of the anatomy and architecture of the breast—a more intuitive anatomically relevant projection.[13–18]

IMAGE REVIEW

Typically, volume ultrasonographic data can be viewed by scrolling through the series of parallel images very quickly; just as with CT series, they can be viewed as a cine loop or can be displayed and reviewed as a complete volume set (interactive cube). Typically the volume sweeps are reviewed as a cine loop. The sweep speed can be adjusted to allow slower review than real-time scanning and, if necessary, frame-by-frame review. Sometimes additional lesions not seen during real-time scanning are detected by the breast imager's review of the volume sets. Now with 3D sonography, there is interactive 3D exploration of pathology and essentially the ability to perform a virtual rescan. Manipulations may include

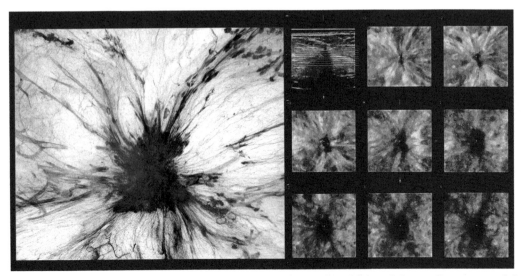

Fig. 20. Three-dimensional subgross histology shows spiculations and straightened Cooper ligaments and ducts as does the coronal image of this small invasive breast cancer.

multiplanar reconstructions, tomographic sections, surface rendering, and so forth to get a different perspective to make a more definitive diagnosis.

Microcalcifications seen on ultrasonography are most easily demonstrated with a cine sweep rather than a static image because microcalcifications are visualized using ultrasonography because of partial voluming and the nature of the surrounding tissue (T. Stavros, personal communication, 2011).

IMAGE ANALYSIS

Image analysis varies between the various vendors and is an area of interest for future product

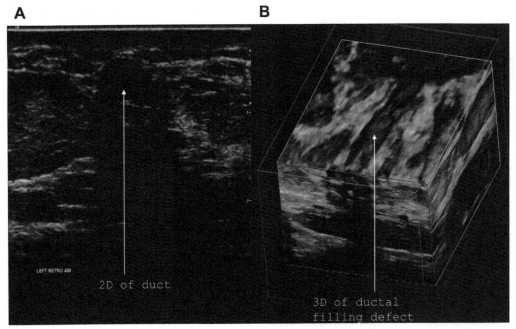

Fig. 21. (A) Acquisition image and (B) coronal reformation. The 2D image demonstrates a round structure that is seen on multiple contiguous images. Sonologists can extrapolate and triangulate in their brain that this represents a distended duct but observe how readily apparent this is when the 3D image is displayed in the coronal plane.

A

B

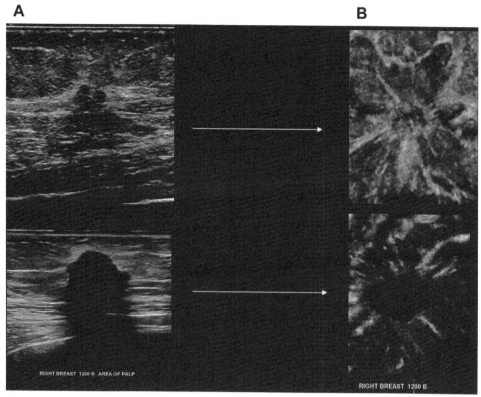

Fig. 22. Breast cancer: coronal plane. (*A*) Acquisition plane and (*B*) coronal plane. Spicules may not always be evident in the 2D image because they are often best demonstrated in the coronal plane. The echogenic halo frequently seen is thought to represent unresolved spiculations or peritumoral edema.

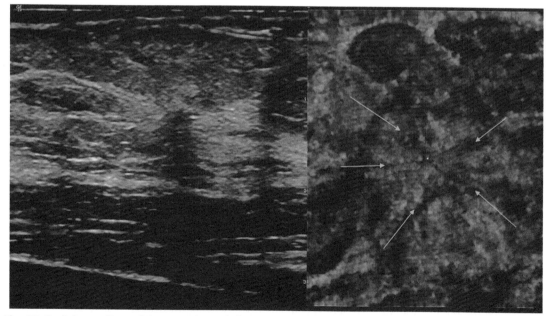

Fig. 23. Radial scar. Coronal images of a radial scar. Acquisition image shows an area of partial shadowing, whereas the coronal image shows spiculation or distortion without a central nidus or nodule (*arrows*).

development. For most clinical situations, direct viewing of the volume data, whether as multiplanar or volume rendered displays, is sufficient. In some situations, that is, the patient on neoadjuvant chemotherapy or short-term follow-up for a probably benign lesion, some form of quantitative analysis is needed. This requirement might represent an automated lesion volume measurement or other forms of quick quantitative analysis. Lesion volumes, especially those with irregular shapes, may be more accurately measured using ultrasonography than traditional 2D ultrasonography. These measurements can assist in therapy monitoring and determination of follow-up intervals. At present, volume measurements are performed by manually tracing the area, which can be time consuming.

APPLICATIONS IN BREAST ULTRASONOGRAPHY

It is difficult to downplay the potential effect that 3D ultrasonography can have in the breast ultrasound practice.[6,7,13–18] Although the greatest applications for this technique are for the indeterminate and malignant-appearing lesions, it is also very helpful to reassure the breast imager on the benign appearance of certain areas and lesions (**Boxes 2** and **3**).

CLINICAL EXAMPLES
Benign

Three-dimensional ultrasonography can play an important role in confirming the benign nature of

---

Box 2
Uses of 3D ultrasonography

1. Determines the greatest tumor dimension and extent of involvement, thus helping to more accurately stage the lesion involvement from an imaging perspective. It can demonstrate ductal extension, tumor bridging, or extension of Cooper ligaments often better than conventional imaging. Volume breast sonography offers unique 3D perspectives on the location, extent, and malignant behavior patterns of breast cancer.
2. Helps the breast imager make diagnoses that are difficult or impossible using 2D imaging; it provides a more confident and accurate diagnosis and serves as a complementary tool to mammography and MRI, helping to increase specificity.
3. Displays pathologic condition in a manner that is more intuitive to our surgical colleagues; it improves detection, staging, determination of extent of disease and helps find multifocal disease thus helping with preoperative planning.
4. Communicates the examination findings to

   a. Surgeons
   b. Referring providers
   c. Patients
   d. Students, residents, fellows

5. Determines which indeterminate lesions should undergo percutaneous biopsy; the additional information from virtually any perspectives is often helpful. Coronal images can now be viewed in a routine fashion, something not possible with 2D ultrasonography. These coronal images often reveal subtle architectural changes that were missed with conventional scanning and influence the decision for tissue sampling.
6. Lessens user variability when measuring lesions or monitoring lesion change on serial examinations (ie, BI-RAD 3 or neoadjuvant follow-up).
7. Shortens the examination time and keeps the breast imager from having to rescan the patient, which prevents delays in the daily schedule and improves the department workflow. The area of interest can be virtually rescanned after the patient has left without loss of diagnostic information.
8. Confirms the benign morphology of questionable lesions or reassures the imager that an area of concern is nothing more than a pseudolesion.
9. Networks with colleagues or experts in the field for their input and opinion. Provides the ability to send 3D packets of information from one site to another.
10. Better evaluates breast mass vascularity.
11. Displays curved ductal structures in a single image with the use of volume-rendering methods of the entire volume.
12. Guides interventional procedures, providing accurate identification of needle/catheter placement (ie, partial breast irradiation catheters) combined with viewing of resliced planes, and rendered images facilitate localization of anatomy and devices within the volume.

frequently encountered lesions and may lend additional insights into intraductal papillary pathology (**Figs. 24–26**).

Malignant

Volume imaging gives us additional perceptional opportunities to detect early breast cancer by identifying either serial images of the altered TDLU or the architectural distortion seen with invasive lesions. It allows us to better understand and visualize the early lesion surface changes and the associated changes in the surrounding mammary and supporting tissues (**Figs. 27** and **28**).

ADVANTAGES

Two-dimensional ultrasonography as currently practiced lacks reproducibility and precision.[5,13–18] Using conventional ultrasonography, sonographers may miss a particular anatomic detail if they cannot see it or if the probe's scanning angle is not right. Unlike CT and MRI, which produce uniform sequential images of anatomy, breast ultrasound examinations differ from clinic to clinic and operator to operator. Three-dimensional or volume sonography is changing this. The result is a series of parallel slices that represent the volume of tissue just scanned, so all the relevant anatomy is saved for review. The ability to see every detail during scanning ceases to be an issue. All the information needed for interpretation is contained in the volume.

Volumetric studies offer several other advantages for the breast imager. As the daily demands stress the limitations of equipment and staff, volume scans are fast; they can improve workflow by allowing the sonographer to scan an area without stopping to take measurements or, in many situations, having to wait for a rescan by the breast imager. This scanning technique makes significant changes in everyday workflow. Because the volume of data has been saved, the breast imager can virtually rescan the area of interest after the patient has left, thus not interrupting the schedule while not sacrificing any diagnostic information. This eliminates the need to rescan. The shortened scan times lead to less stress-related injuries for staff and additional time for add-on examinations. This improved productivity boosts the bottom line and allows providers to accommodate a growing number of studies without the need for additional staff or equipment. By providing dynamic information, the ability to manipulate the data to view the area of interest in any planes, volumetric ultrasonography, allows the breast imagers to be more confident in their diagnosis and treatment recommendations. These examinations are also less user dependent because the volume sweeps allow the reviewer to see what the sonographer saw without actually being there. You can reconstruct the information and navigate through it long after the patient has gone.

In addition, volume scanning helps reduce unnecessary patient anxiety by reducing the time

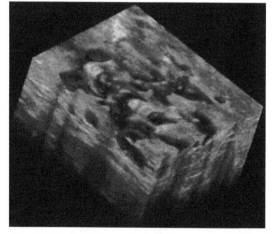

Fig. 24. Coronal image: ductal ectasia. Coronal imaging is helpful in evaluating ductal pathologic condition because of the fact that the major ducts lie in the coronal plane (parallel orientation).

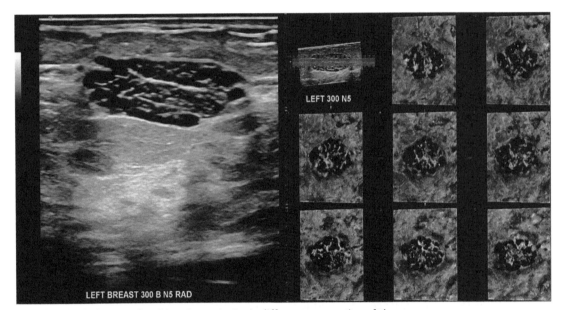

Fig. 25. Coronal images of multicystic areas give a different perspective of the same process.

it takes to get on the department's schedule because of reduced scheduling backlog and also frequently eliminates waiting partially dressed in an examination room while the sonographer checks the scan with the supervising breast imager (see **Box 2**). This technique often eliminates the need to rescan, and, frequently, reconstruction by the sonographer on the units instantly relieves the patient's anxiety, such as showing the patient that the abnormality she is feeling is nothing more than the valve of her saline implant. It frequently simplifies confusing anatomy

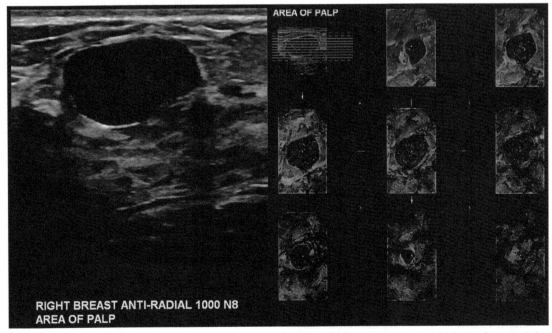

Fig. 26. Fibroadenomas when displayed in the coronal plane still have benign morphologic characteristics; however, they may exhibit additional lobulations from this perspective.

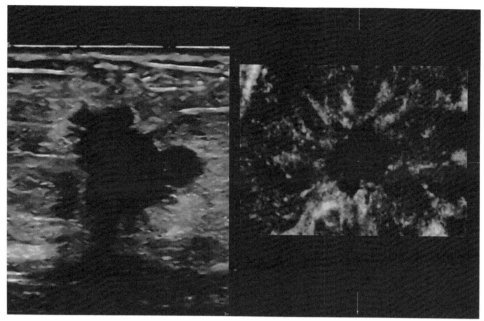

Fig. 27. Coronal images of suspicious 2D images show distortion (retraction) in the coronal plane.

into a plane or projection that is more easily under-stood by the patient, referring physician or consulting breast surgeon (**Fig. 29**).

Sonographers and breast imagers find this technology very gratifying in that the sonographer now spends more time talking to the patients, less stressed as they are not continually behind by the delays in waiting for the breast imager to rescan. Also, volume ultrasonography helps address a major concern in the profession, that is, work-related repetitive stress injuries. Several studies have shown a reduction in repetitive stress injuries using this technique.

Another advantage of the 3D reconstructions is that they can be downloaded and sent to the referring physicians and demand far less interpretive

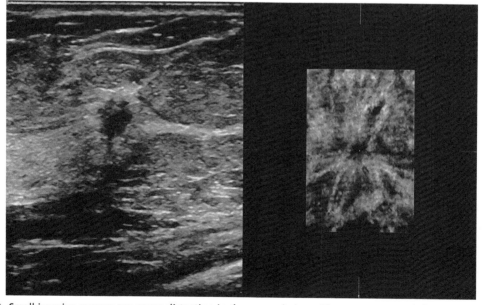

Fig. 28. Small invasive cancers can cause distortion in the coronal plane. I have seen coronal distortion in lesions smaller than 5 mm in size.

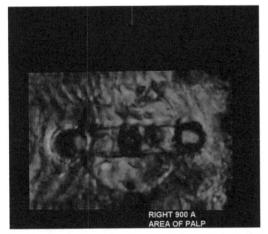

RIGHT 900 A
AREA OF PALP

Fig. 29. Three-dimensional coronal image of a palpable breast lump in a young patient with a saline implant. The coronal image demonstrates that the palpable region corresponds to the implant valve.

skills from the receiving physician than do 2D images or traditional cine sweeps of ultrasound examinations. The reconstructed images provide images that are more akin to standard Netter illustrations and often make a difference in diagnosis. The 3D images are often more intuitive to our surgical colleagues and are immensely helpful when planning breast conservation surgery or oncoplastic procedures. It is also helpful when they are explaining the anticipated procedures to the patient.

Three-dimensional imaging has given the breast imager a whole new level of important diagnostic information by providing the ability to study a breast mass, its vascularity, and the surrounding tissue in 3 orthogonal planes. In breast imaging, 3D imaging has given new insights into tumor growth patterns. Each cancer can now be more accurately measured (size) and tumoral margins

defined. Tumor extensions can be displayed and satellite lesions demonstrated. Multifocal breast cancer is common. Translating and rotating the acquired 3D volume data of a breast cancer and the surrounding tissue make the underlying process of multifocal disease easier to demonstrate and understand. All these factors have improved our diagnostic capabilities while helping us to more accurately stage these cancers. It also allows us to quantitatively determine the success of our treatments when following patients by demonstrating subtle changes in the volume of tumor masses (**Fig. 30**).

DISADVANTAGES/LIMITATIONS

Like any imaging modality there are limitations and disadvantages to the techniques. A robust PACS system with advanced visualization capability or an independent ultrasonographic workstation is required to properly view and interpret volume scans because most schedules do not allow time to render, display, and manipulate these studies on the machine console. Large lesions present a problem for the field of view (FOV) of calibrated 3D probes; the hand-held volume sweeps are less affected by the size of the lesion. There are certain technical challenges that must be overcome to integrate into the daily routine. Details of these challenges are beyond the scope of this article, but the reader should note that these are large data sets and like CT and MRI require close cooperation with your information technology department. The Digital Imaging and Communications in Medicine (DICOM) standard continues to evolve with recently released DICOM standards for archiving 3D/4D ultrasound images. Many vendors have DICOM tags, which make interpretation and display limited to nonproprietary systems. There is no rationale for PACS systems to remain

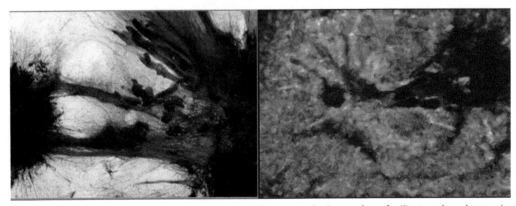

Fig. 30. Multifocal breast cancers are common, and the coronal plane often facilitates the observation of bridging ductal structures distended with ductal carcinoma in situ. (*Courtesy of* Dr Laszlo Tabar, Falun, Sweden.)

confined to the realm of 2D imaging while plug-ins or add-ons software handles 3D imaging. Integration of 3D with PACS is a key area of current vendor product development.

This integration is not a costly investment, and the cost can be recouped in a short time with the increased revenue from the additional examinations you are now able to perform. Ultrasound BI-RADS was developed for 2D ultrasonography, and, now with the additional information available with 3D imaging, imagers find themselves looking for appropriate descriptors to describe and characterize the additional findings encountered. Also, some of the old rules such as 2 or 3 gentle lobulations for Cat. 3 lesions are not applicable because the same lesion is now shown to have 6 to 8 gentle lobulations when viewing from multiple planes and viewing perspectives. The BI-RADS committee has recognized this dilemma and is working on standardizing the descriptors between mammography, breast ultrasonography, and breast MRI.

With any new service, there needs to be a quality control program to assure consistency and accuracy of the examinations. We addressed this by establishing a super user (a trusted senior breast sonographer) position to review each study and assist the staff in the learning process. Consistent results come from a team effort in which education and constant learning as well as staff development are top priorities.

WORKFLOW ISSUES

Depending on the size of breast ultrasound section, it may be necessary to modify your workflow to accommodate the additional patient load and scan volumes.[4–6,21] Many centers have adapted volume sonography by necessity, others for the diagnostic confidence it offers. There are many workflow options depending on the specifics of your individual breast center, which will depend on the number of ultrasound machines, staff, and the typical workflow scenarios in your department. Three-dimensional ultrasonography can be time consuming for the breast imager, and there is a learning curve; however, when working closely with our staff, we made several modifications, which clearly emphasized the overall improvement in our workflow efficiency.

As imaging numbers increase, it is no longer possible to rescan every patient. This concept is foreign for many breast imagers who feel they must scan every patient. Volume sonography allows to significantly improve efficiency without compromising quality. In reality, it is a more efficient method of acquiring optimal 2D images. Volume imaging offers huge advantages in the way imagers work. The present medical environment demands consistency, accuracy, and efficient workflow.

ARTIFACTS: PITFALLS

Because current processing involves user-defined parameters, such as slice thickness and interslice spacing, which affects reconstruction voxel dimensions, there is opportunity to remove vital information and to distort the appearance of a lesion or to create pseudolesions through partial voluming. Three-dimensional sonography like any imaging modality has its own set of unique artifacts that one must be aware of to avoid misinterpretation of appearance. Correct identification of these artifacts is essential because artifacts may mimic masses because of acoustic dropout or shadowing. These artifacts are initially more difficult to recognize because of the different and unfamiliar displays. Rendering can also introduce artifacts. Two-dimensional artifacts are also problematic at times because the 3D image is built from serial 2D images. Viewing the source images as well as acquiring from multiple orientations may avoid some artifacts (D. Pretorius, personal communication, 2010).

PUTTING THIS ALL TOGETHER

Ultrasonography has always been an extremely versatile breast imaging modality because of its ability to scan the internal structures of the breast in a noninvasive and cost-effective manner. The technique is unique in its ability to image patient anatomy and physiology in real time. With the introduction of volume sonography, the breast imager now has ways to further display and interrogate breast pathology not possible with some of the other traditional breast imaging techniques.

In breast ultrasonography, like other ultrasound examinations, the quality of the examination is based largely on the experience and skill of the person obtaining the images. Understandably, this leads to a more frequent need or desire for breast imagers to perform their own additional imaging after the sonographer's examination. However, with the demands of the current breast center and the increasing volumes of patients, additional imaging is not always possible, which leads to disruption of the daily scan schedule, patient recalls, and, ultimately, anxious patients.

Three-dimensional ultrasonography as described depends less on the operator and introduces new flexibility into the breast center schedule while not compromising on the diagnostic quality of the examination. The breast imager can now reconstruct volume in any plane regardless of the acquisition plane and essentially allows the physicians interpreting the scan to review the entire volume as though they were actually scanning the patients themselves. These efficiencies, flexibilities, and multiplanar reconstructions are similar to those that have been used in CT and MRI for several years.[22]

Considering the factors in **Box 4**, our entire breast scanning protocols were revised to include volume acquisitions in 2005, and these protocols have been used as part of our routine examination since that time.

Each breast center is unique, so I describe how our center implemented these changes and how we use volume ultrasonography in our daily practices. We standardized all the equipments, workstations, and scanning protocols; our goal was to address the patient volumes (backlog of anxious patients), save our valued staff from repetitive injuries, and eliminate the need for physician rescan while not compromising examination diagnostic quality or accuracy.

In our center, we perform whole breast ultrasonography on mammography or clinically detected abnormalities and reserve a focused examination to those patients referred for short-term follow-up (BI-RADS 3).

We routinely sweep (free-hand volume acquisition)

1. The reason for examination
   a. Abnormal mammogram
      i. Masslike asymmetries
      ii. Focal asymmetry
      iii. Microcalcifications
      iv. Architectural distortion
   b. Abnormal clinical examination result
      i. Palpable nodules/masses
      ii. Nipple inversion/change
      iii. Gynecomastia
      iv. Mastitis/breast abscess

   c. Abnormal symptoms
      i. Focal pain/tenderness
      ii. Nipple discharge
2. Any solid mass or complex cystic lesion encountered during examination
3. Any ductal pathology (ie, papillomas)
4. Implant complications
5. Specific entities or anatomic areas where pathology is hard to adequately demonstrate with static images
   a. Retroareolar and axillary regions
   b. Scars
6. When it is important to demonstrate anatomic and spatial relationships
   a. Relation of lesion to nipple
   b. Implant capsule continuity
   c. Seroma to scar
   d. Multifocal lesions
   e. Ductal filling defect in relation to nipple
7. Any area of sonographer concern.

Our goal is to avoid the breast imager having to rescan by completely documenting the abnormality or lesion. All suspicious findings are discussed and reviewed with the breast imager before letting the patient leave. The patients requiring tissue sampling (biopsy) are scheduled before they leave the department.

3D Calibrated Probe: Automatic Volume Acquisition

Evaluation with the dedicated 3D breast transducer to suspicious areas identified during the routine breast examinations is reserved, realizing that there is a limited FOV with this transducer. This evaluation has been found very helpful in assessing the following because they reduce operator dependence and allow for consistent results:

a. Nipple discharge and the retroareolar regions in patients with ductal ectasia, gynecomastia, or intraductal filling defects
b. Microcalcifications
c. Atypical cysts
d. Solid masses
e. Architectural distortion.

The data sets that are obtained are very large and require additional time to transfer to the workstations. In general, the 3D images produced are consistently excellent, the major limitations being the size of the transducer for small-handed sonographers or breast imagers and the fact that you must switch to another transducer to obtain these images.

We typically use both techniques on almost every breast ultrasound examination. We feel

---

Box 4
Reasons that breast lesions (pathology) are missed

- Use of old equipment (poor image quality/resolution)
- The ultrasound image not optimized to enhance lesion conspicuity
- Perceptual error (breast imager did not see or recognize abnormality)
- Examination performed as a focused examination (the lesion was not scanned)
- Lesion not visible on ultrasonography

that there are advantages and limitations to both techniques, and the best examinations come from optimizing the strengths of both.

SUMMARY

Given the 3D nature of our body organs, the 3D applications in general ultrasonography are limitless. The applications of this technique in pelvis/obstetric and cardiac imaging have set new standards in these fields, and, as such, volume (3D) ultrasonography offers a new paradigm in breast ultrasonography. For years, images of organs and pathology have been taken in 2 planes; however, there is much to be learned beyond these 2 planes. In breast imaging, volume ultrasonography allows a unique and diagnostic view of breast pathology. The technique allows better visualization of complex structures and their relationships to surrounding structures, increasing our diagnostic confidence. The greatest applications of the technique are probably in characterizing the morphologic features and extent of malignant lesions. Volume ultrasonography frequently demonstrates 1 to 2 additional findings that change either the BI-RADS classification or lesion size, both of which affect subsequent surgical or interventional planning. The technique also gives the breast imager reassurance in diagnosing benign processes encountered in daily scanning. As technology advances, the detail, speed, and clinical applications continue to broaden. Volume sonography, elastography, and contrast-enhanced ultrasonography are poised to give the breast center new and more effective diagnostic tool. These tools will change the way you image the breast with ultrasound (a fresh new look), by changing the way you acquire, review and interpret breast ultrasound examinations – it offers diagnostic opportunities not readily available with 2D imaging.

There is ongoing research in many areas of future applications (ie, contrast, gene therapy, and so forth). We have just begun to explore the various ways 3D ultrasound will impact our daily lives and practices. It allows you to look at data from another perspective. It broadens our knowledge and our ways of reaching diagnosis in complex lesions and hopefully this will help us tailor our treatment to the patient.

Three-dimensional breast ultrasonography is a powerful tool for the breast imager that has the potential much like breast MRI to profoundly affect the care of our patients with breast cancer. It is also an integral part of the technology solution to our workflow issues. There are both clinical and financial benefits for the department. It is

transforming both patient evaluation and management. There are continued advances, and the technique continues to evolve with further refinements in image resolution because the vendors apply more powerful processors in association with improved transducer technology, multiple display options, and expansion of applications. Imagers will have to be asked—what have we been missing? Imagers will find that volume (3D) sonography will make them a better 2D imager because they will now look for subtle architectural changes they once passed over and that having entered into the 3D world of ultrasonography, there is no going back. Welcome to the new world of breast ultrasonography!

ACKNOWLEDGMENTS

I would like to acknowledge and thank the following individuals for their input, mentoring, and patience in my 3D learning experience: Laszlo Tabar, MD, and Thomas Stavros, MD; Janice Whyte, RDMS, and our sonography staff; and Kelli Bultman, RDMS, and J.P. Moreland, BS, RDMS, GE Healthcare.

REFERENCES

1. Kelly K, Dean J, Comulada WS, et al. Breast cancer detection using automated whole breast ultrasound and mammography in radiographically dense breast. Eur Radiol 2010;20:734–42.
2. Lander M, Tabar L. Automated 3-D breast ultrasound as a promising adjunctive screening tool for examining the dense portion of the breast, in press.
3. Daher N. 3D imaging increases clinical relevance. 2007;60–2. Available at: TNonline.net. Accessed November, 2007.
4. Brandli L. Benefits of protocol driven ultrasound exams. Radiol Manage 2007;29(4):56–9, 1–4.
5. Garra B, Doherty J. Advanced applications make ultrasound more competitive. Diagn Imag 2008 [online].
6. Barnes E. Medical image processing has room to grow. Parts 1, 23. Tucson (AZ): Aunt Minnie; 2006.
7. Tabar L, Tot T, Dean P. Practical breast pathology. New York (NY): Thieme Publishing; 2002.
8. Watermann D, Foldi M, Hanjalic-Beck A, et al. Three dimensional ultrasound for the assessment of breast lesions. Ultrasound Obstet Gynecol 2005;25:592–8.
9. Zhou S, Zeng W, Fan Y, et al. Does the "Sun Sign" on coronal plane and 3D ultrasound imaging aid the accurate diagnosis of breast lesions? JUIM 2009;35:S126.
10. Lazebnik R, Desser T. Clinical 3D ultrasound imaging: beyond obstetrical applications. Diagn Imag 2007;1–5 [online].
11. Stavros AT. Breast ultrasound. Philadelphia (PA): Lippincott Williamson & Wilkins; 2004.

12. Tabar L, Tot T, Dean P. Breast cancer, the art and science of early detection with mammography. New York (NY): Thieme Publishing; 2005.

13. Benacerraf B. Three-dimensional ultrasound of the fetus. Is it necessary? Waukesha (WI): GE Publications; 2006.

14. Bultman K. VIP multicenter study, 30% less scan time. Waukesha (WI): GE Publications; 2006.

15. Dahiya N. The basics of 3D/4D ultrasound. Waukesha (WI): GE Publications; 2005.

16. McDonald D, Bultman K. Volume US and VIP in breast imaging. Waukesha (WI): GE Publications; 2005.

17. VIP: volume imaging protocol for LOGIC9, LOGIC 7 and LOGICworks. Waukesha (WI): GE Publications; 2010.

18. Weismann CF. 3D/4D ultrasound breast imaging. Waukesha (WI): GE Publications; 2007.

19. Graziano L. Mechanics in tumor growth. In: Francesco M, Luigi P, Rajagopal KR, editors. Modeling of biological materials. Boston (MA): Birkhauser; 2007. p. 267–328.

20. Tessler F, Brown J. Volume ultrasound competes with multiplanar CT and MRI. Diagn Imag 2007; 81–6 [online].

21. Bicknell SG, Hagel J. Impact of 3-D sonography on workroom time efficiency. AJR Am J Roentgenol 2007;188:966–9.

22. Benacerraff B, Shipp T, Bromley B. Three-dimensional US of the fetus: volume imaging. Radiology 2006;238(3):988–96.

Ultrasound Elastography of Breast Lesions

Christopher Comstock, MD

KEYWORDS

• Ultrasound elastography • Lesion • Elasticity • Shear wave

Since the inception of breast ultrasonography, lesion compressibility has often been subjectively assessed during real-time scanning using manual compression (**Fig. 1**). In general, benign processes are often soft and mobile, whereas malignant conditions tend to be hard or firm. However, the process of evaluating lesion compressibility or stiffness on ultrasound (US) elastography and the incorporation of such data into diagnostic decision making have not been standardized. Static or compressive elastography (US strain imaging) and acoustic radiation force impulse (ARFI), of which shear wave elastography is a subtype, are the 2 main methods of breast US elastography that have emerged and they differ by the type of stress or vibration applied. The goal of both these methods is to provide a standardized elastography process and an objective representation of lesion stiffness to improve diagnostic confidence and increase specificity of the US interpretation. However, although malignant lesions tend to be stiffer than benign lesions, exceptions such as mucinous carcinomas, necrotic tumors, and high-grade carcinomas may potentially lead to false-negative results. In addition, benign conditions that are firm or stiff, such as scarring, fibrosis, and complex fibroadenomas, may be misinterpreted as malignant. Therefore, elastography information alone should not be used for lesion analysis but rather as an adjunct to the standard gray-scale morphologic and color Doppler information.

BASIC PRINCIPLES OF ELASTOGRAPHY

Tissue stiffness or elasticity can be measured by a physical quantity called the Young modulus and expressed in pressure units, that is, pascal or, more commonly, kilopascal. The relationship between the applied external stress and induced strain is expressed in the Young modulus as the ratio between the applied stress and the induced strain (**Fig. 2**). Typical values of elasticity in various tissue types have been reported in the literature (**Table 1**). The basic process of US elastography involves inducing some form of stress in the tissue (low-frequency vibration), imaging the tissue before and after the stress, and then analyzing the deformation (strain) of lesions. Tissue deformation between the prestress and poststress images is calculated by various spectral tracking or A-line pair cross-correlation methods.[1] The US Food and Drug Administration has not approved quantitation of elasticity, so the degree of tissue deformation is represented in relative terms through color overlay maps (elastogram) applied to the standard gray-scale image. The color spectrum for the overlay maps have not been standardized among vendors, but, in general, for compressive elastography, red indicates softer regions and blue indicates more firm areas. The reverse color scheme has been used for shear wave color maps. Both the color and pattern of the elastogram may give clues about the type of lesion being interrogated. General

Breast Imaging Service, Department of Radiology, Memorial Sloan-Kettering Cancer Center, 1275 York Avenue, New York, NY 10065, USA
E-mail address: ComstocC@mskcc.org

Ultrasound Clin 6 (2011) 407–415
doi:10.1016/j.cult.2011.05.004
1556-858X/11/$ – see front matter © 2011 Published by Elsevier Inc.

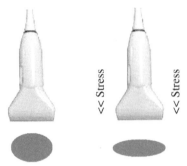

Fig. 1. Evaluation of compressibility during real-time gray-scale ultrasonography. A subjective assessment of a lesion's compressibility (stiffness) can be performed during real-time US scanning by applying manual compression with the transducer. Compressive or static elastography involves very light repeated manual compression and a US unit capable of measuring the tissue deformation from the precompression and postcompression images.

Table 1 Relative values of elasticity in different types of tissues		
Types of Soft Tissue		Young Modulus (Elasticity in kPa)
Breast	Normal fat	18–24
	Normal glandular	28–66
	Fibrous tissue	96–244
	Carcinoma	22–560
Prostate	Normal gland	55–71
	Benign prostatic hyperplasia	36–41
	Carcinoma	96–241
Liver	Normal	0.4–6
	Cirrhosis	15–100

elastogram patterns, in terms of homogeneity, size, and shape, include monochromatic (homogeneous with the lesion clearly visible beneath overlay), nearly homogeneous, and heterogeneous (both soft and hard colors extending into the periphery of the lesion) patterns. The pattern and depiction of the elastogram may be specific to the particular elastography method being used. The quantitation method may also involve the placement of regions of interest in normal tissue, such as subcutaneous fat, whereby stiffness ratios of lesion to background can be calculated. Factors that may affect the elastography include the size and depth of the lesion as well as the angle of the US transducer. Elasticity information should be considered along with the gray-scale morphologic characteristics of the lesion.

STATIC OR COMPRESSIVE ELASTOGRAPHY

In static or compression elastography, stress is applied by repeated light manual compression of

$$E = \frac{s}{e} = \frac{\text{Applied stress}}{\text{Induced strain}}$$

Fig. 2. The Young modulus is a measure of the stiffness of an elastic material. The Young modulus or elasticity (E) can be calculated by dividing the applied external stress or force (s) by the induced strain or deformation (e). Hard tissue has a higher elasticity than soft tissue.

the transducer on the breast surface resulting in mild deformation of the underlying tissues. Because the compression applied by the user cannot be quantified, the Young modulus cannot be calculated. The amount of lesion deformation can only be depicted as a ratio to normal tissues or displayed in relative terms in gray scale (Fig. 3) or in color (Fig. 4). Early researchers of compressive elastography (Itoh and colleagues[3]) proposed a 5-pattern elastogram scale of increasing suspicion (Fig. 5). In addition to the 5-pattern elastogram scale, the lesion to background elasticity ratio and the elastogram to gray-scale lesion size ratio have been evaluated. It has been postulated that the elastograms of cancers tend to be larger than the corresponding gray-scale images because of surrounding tissue edema and desmoplastic reaction.[4,5] Because of the overlap of the elastographic features of some cancers with benign lesions, morphologically highly suspicious lesions require biopsy, despite an apparently benign elastogram. Elastography may be most useful in evaluation of probably benign or low-suspicion lesions (Fig. 6).

ARFI (SHEAR WAVE ELASTOGRAPHY)

Another form of elastography being used in the breast is called shear wave elastography or shear wave imaging. Unlike compression elastography, in which the stress is applied by the user and may be variable, shear wave elastography uses the acoustic radiation force induced by the US beam itself to perturb the underlying tissue. This force induces mechanical waves, including shear waves, which propagate transversely in the tissue (Fig. 7). Because of the limitation of possible transducer

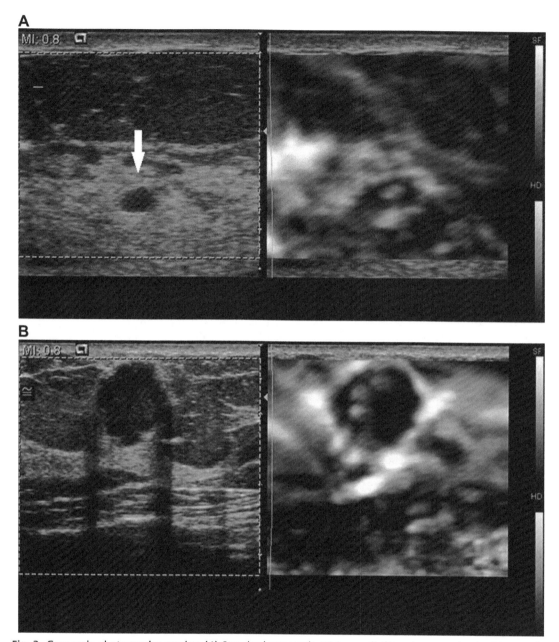

Fig. 3. Gray-scale elastography overlay. (*A*) Standard gray-scale US image (*left*) and gray-scale elasticity overlay (*right*) demonstrating a typical bull's-eye pattern (a rim of high elasticity is seen surrounding an area of central low elasticity) of a benign cyst (*arrow*). (*B*) Ductal carcinoma demonstrating high elasticity (dark areas on the elastogram) as compared with the surrounding tissue. (*Courtesy of* Siemens; with permission.)

heating, US-generated shear waves must be very weak, amounting to only a few micrometers of displacement that dissipates after only a few millimeters of propagation. Shear waves typically propagate in tissue at speeds between 1 and 10 m/s (corresponding to tissue elasticity from 1 to 300 kPa). At this speed, they cross a standard US image field of view in 10 to 20 milliseconds. To

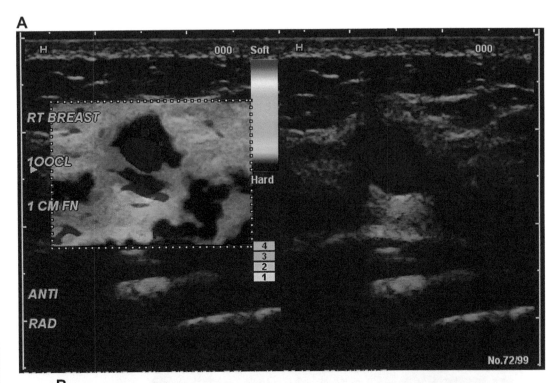

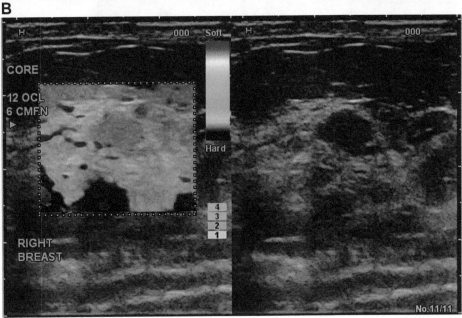

Fig. 4. Compressive elastography clinical images with color overlay (obtained using VISION 8500 SonoElastography [Hitachi Medical Systems America, Inc, Twinsburg, OH, USA]). (*A*) Typical trilaminar color pattern of a benign cyst. The trilaminar pattern (*layers of blue, green, and red*) seen in cysts is believed to be an artifact from aliasing of the color scale.[2] (*B*) Benign fibroadenoma showing a mostly homogeneously soft to medium (*green*) color pattern. (*C*) Invasive ductal carcinoma demonstrating a predominately firm (*blue*) color pattern with extension of the elastogram into the surrounding tissue reaction (*light blue*). (*D*) Benign lipoma (*arrow*) showing a predominately soft color pattern.

C

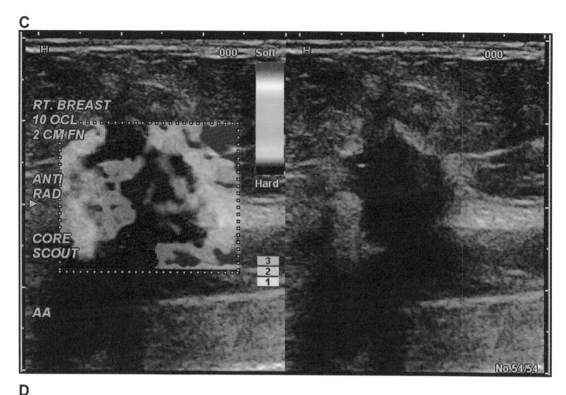

D

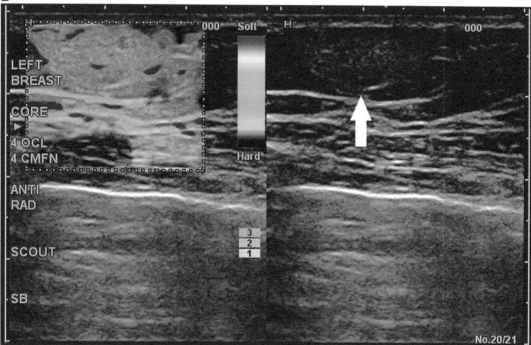

Fig. 4. (*continued*)

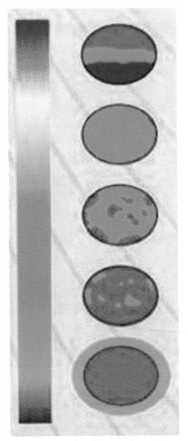

1. Trilaminar - Predominantly liquid

2. Predominantly soft

3. Mixed pattern

4. Predominantly firm

5. Firm, larger than apparent size

Fig. 5. Elastogram color pattern scale. The 5-point color pattern scale for classification of lesions seen on elastography, with 1 being the most benign and 5 being the most suspicious: (1) fluid pattern (trilaminar color pattern), (2) predominantly soft, (3) mixed stiffness (2-color pattern), (4) predominantly firm, and (5) firm with apparent enlargement of lesion on elastography compared with the conventional gray-scale image. (*Modified from* Scaperrotta G, Ferranti C, Costa C, et al. Role of sonoelastography in nonpalpable breast lesions. Eur Radiol 2008;18(11):2383; with permission.)

capture shear waves in sufficient detail, imaging frame rates on the order of several thousand frames per second are required. Recent advances in computer and graphics processing have made possible shear wave imaging by allowing imaging frame rates as high as 20,000 Hz. Because the amount of applied stress is known, shear wave–based elastography is able to provide quantitative elastic information in real time. The stiffer the tissue, the faster the shear wave propagates. As with compression elastography, depending on the nature of the lesion, various stiffness patterns can be seen with shear wave imaging. However, these patterns may be somewhat different from those of manual compression elastography because of the

different forces being measured and the differences in imaging methods (**Fig. 8**).

CLINICAL STUDIES

Multiple studies have been published evaluating the possible role of US elastography in improving the accuracy of breast ultrasonography. Analyses have evaluated various parameters such as the elastogram to gray-scale lesion size ratio, background to lesion elasticity ratio, elastogram pattern, as well as maximal and mean absolute elasticity values in kilopascals (ARFI). Sensitivities of 70% to 96% and specificities of 24% to 90% have been reported.[6–18] Differences in criteria

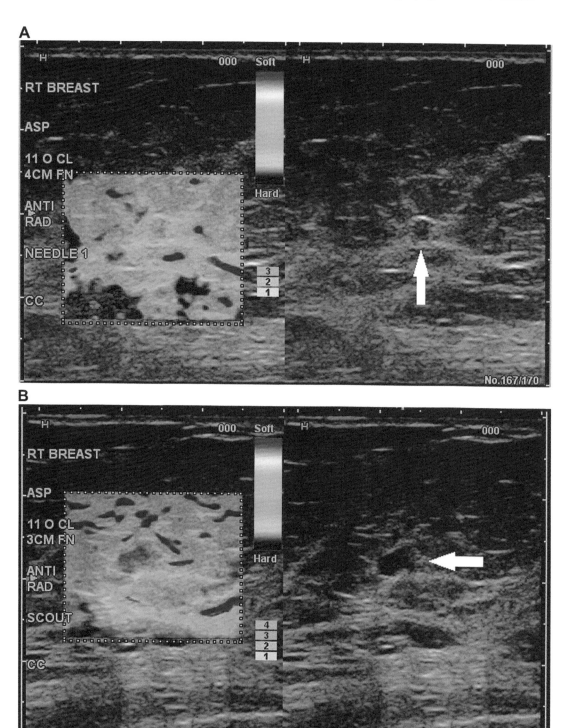

Fig. 6. Potential utility of elastography. Two small hypoechoic structures (*arrows*) seen on gray-scale imaging were initially thought to represent benign complicated cysts. However, elastography demonstrates that they differ in elasticity, with one (*B*) showing a predominately firm (*blue*) color pattern. Biopsy revealed ductal carcinoma in situ. The smaller lesion showing softer elasticity (*A*) proved to be a cyst on aspiration.

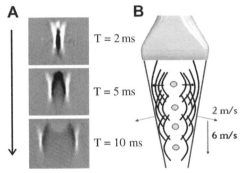

Fig. 7. Propagation of shear waves. (*A*) Phantom images capturing the shear wave propagating lateral to the direction of the applied compression (*arrow*). (*B*) Speed of propagation of the shear wave laterally is approximately 2 m/s. (*Courtesy of* SuperSonic Imagine; with permission.)

for benign/malignant differentiation in these studies may account for some of the variability in results. However, the variability is also in part because of the biologic heterogeneity of benign and cancerous lesions. Cancers with soft features, such as mucinous carcinoma, high-grade cancers, and cancers with necrosis, may potentially cause false-negative results on elastography alone. Conversely, fibroadenomas with high cellularity, marked stromal fibrosis, and complex fibroadenomas tend to be harder and may have elastographic features similar to carcinomas.[19] Elastography has been helpful in elucidating the benign nature of complicated cysts, hematomas, and atypical-appearing fibroadenomas.[20,21] A 17-site worldwide multicenter clinical trial evaluating shear wave elastography is currently underway. Initial

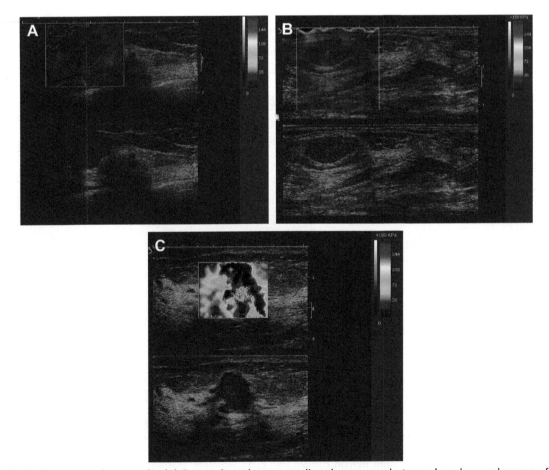

Fig. 8. Shear wave elastography. (*A*) Gray-scale and corresponding shear wave elastography color overlay map of a simple cyst. The cyst is seen to have a black void on the elasticity image. (*B*) A benign fibroadenoma demonstrates a homogeneously soft pattern (*blue*) on the elasticity image. (*C*) Invasive ductal carcinoma demonstrating a firm high-elasticity pattern (*red*) that is larger than the corresponding gray-scale lesion size. An elastogram that is larger than the gray-scale lesion size is suspicious and may relate to stiffening of the surrounding tissue as a result of edema and desmoplastic reaction. (*Courtesy of* SuperSonic Imagine; with permission.)

results seem to indicate reproducibility as well as improved diagnostic accuracy with shear wave elastography.

SUMMARY

The addition of stiffness as a lesion feature, in combination with other lesion parameters, may help to increase the diagnostic confidence and accuracy of breast ultrasonography. The most useful application of elastography may be in reducing the number of short-term follow-ups (BI-RADS [Breast Imaging Reporting and Data System] 3) of probably benign masses, biopsies of low-suspicion benign masses, and aspirations of borderline or complicated cysts. The elastographic information should not be used to avoid biopsy of a morphologically highly suspicious mass or clinically suspicious mass. Further prospective clinical trials are needed to better define its optimal use and determine which parameters are most predictive. In addition, elastography descriptors need to be standardized and incorporated into future American College of Radiology Breast Ultrasound BI-RADS Lexicon editions. The clinical use of elastography will undoubtedly continue to grow because most vendors now offer US units with elastography as an option.

REFERENCES

1. Ophir J, Céspedes I, Ponnekanti H, et al. Elastography: a quantitative method for imaging the elasticity of biological tissues. Ultrason Imaging 1991;13(2): 111–34.
2. Cho N, Moon WK, Chang JM, et al. Aliasing artifact depicted on ultrasound (US)-elastography for breast cystic lesions mimicking solid masses. Acta Radiol 2011;52:3–7.
3. Itoh A, Ueno E, Tohno E, et al. Breast disease: clinical application of US elastography for diagnosis. Radiology 2006;239:341–50.
4. Garra BS, El Cespedes, Ophir J, et al. Elastography of breast lesions: initial clinical results. Radiology 1997;202:79–86.
5. Hall TJ, Zhu Y, Spalding CS. In vivo real-time freehand palpation imaging. Ultrasound Med Biol 2003;29:427–35.
6. Scaperrotta G, Ferranti C, Costa C, et al. Role of sonoelastography in non-palpable breast lesions. Eur Radiol 2008;18:2381–9.
7. Burnside ES, Hall TJ, Sommer AM, et al. Differentiating benign from malignant solid breast masses with US strain imaging. Radiology 2007;245:401–10.
8. FleuryEde F, Fleury JC, Piato S, et al. New elastographic classification of breast lesions during and after compression. Diagn Interv Radiol 2009;15: 96–103.
9. Tardivon A, El Khoury C, Thibault F, et al. Elastography of the breast: a prospective study of 122 lesions. J Radiol 2007;88:657–62 [in French].
10. Zhi H, Ou B, Luo BM, et al. Comparison of ultrasound elastography, mammography, and sonography in the diagnosis of solid breast lesions. J Ultrasound Med 2007;26:807–15.
11. Schaefer FK, Heer I, Schaefer PJ, et al. Breast ultrasound elastography - results of 193 breast lesions in a prospective study with histopathologic correlation. Eur J Radiol 2011;77:450–6.
12. Regini E, Bagnera S, Tota D, et al. Role of sonoelastography in characterising breast nodules. Preliminary experience with 120 lesions. Radiol Med 2010;115:551–62.
13. Regner DM, Hesley GK, Hangiandreou NJ, et al. Breast lesions: evaluation with US strain imaging—clinical experience of multiple observers. Radiology 2006;238:425–37.
14. Moon WK, Huang C-S, Shen W-C, et al. Analysis of elastographic and B-mode features at sonoelastography for breast tumor classification. Ultrasound Med Biol 2009;35:1794–802.
15. Zhu QL, Jiang YX, Liu JB, et al. Real-time ultrasound elastography: its potential role in assessment of breast lesions. Ultrasound Med Biol 2008; 34:1232–8.
16. Thomas A, Fischer T, Frey H, et al. Real-time elastography—an advanced method of ultrasound: first results in 108 patients with breast lesions. Ultrasound Obstet Gynecol 2006;28:335–40.
17. Sohn YM, Kim MJ, Kim EK, et al. Sonographic elastography combined with conventional sonography: how much is it helpful for diagnostic performance? J Ultrasound Med 2009;28:413–20.
18. Athanasiou A, Tardivon A, Tanter M, et al. Breast lesions: quantitative elastography with supersonic shear imaging—preliminary results. Radiology 2010; 256:297–303.
19. Fleury EF, Rinaldi JF, Piato S, et al. Appearance of breast masses on sonoelastography with special focus on the diagnosis of fibroadenomas. Eur Radiol 2009;19:1337–46.
20. Booi RC, Carson PL, O'Donnell M, et al. Characterization of cysts using differential correlation coefficient values from two dimensional breast elastography: preliminary study. Ultrasound Med Biol 2008;34: 12–21.
21. Ginat DT, Destounis SV, Barr RG, et al. US elastography of breast and prostate lesions. Radiographics 2009;29:2007–16.

Index

Note: Page numbers of article titles are in **boldface** type.

A

Acoustic radiation force impulse elastography,
  408–409, 412
Adenopathy, silicone, 362–363
Alveolar lobular carcinoma, 314
Angio map, in three-dimensional ultrasonography,
  387

B

Background noise, reduction of, 302–306
Barrier disruption, in implants, 358–359
Beamforming, digital, 300
Biopsy
  advantages of, 327
  history of, 327
  methods for, 330–331
  of calcifications, 337–342
  of lymph nodes
    in invasive lobular carcinoma, 320–321
    percutaneous, 377–378
    sentinel, 376–377
  procedure for, **327–333**
  sensitivity of, 330–331
Breast ultrasound
  elastography, 301, 308–310, **407–415**
  for biopsy. *See* Biopsy.
  for implants, **345–368**
  lymph node imaging and, **369–380**
  physics and technology of, **313–325**
    computer-aided diagnosis, 310
    Doppler, 308
    speckle reduction, 302–306
    speed of sound correction, 302
    system architecture, 300–302
    tissue elasticity, 308–310
    tissue harmonic imaging, 306–308
  physics of, **299–312**
  three-dimensional, **381–406**
Breast-specific gamma imaging, 323

C

Calcifications
  biopsy of, 337–342
  evaluation of, 335–337
  in implants, 346
  in invasive lobular carcinoma, 316–317
  mammography for, 335–336

Cancer

Cancer
  biopsy for. *See* Biopsy.
  elastography for, **407–415**
  invasive lobular carcinoma, **313–325**
  metastasis from. *See* Metastasis.
  three-dimensional ultrasonography for, **381–406**
Carcinoma, invasive lobular. *See* Invasive lobular
  carcinoma.
Coded excitation technology, 300
Compression (static) elastography, 408, 410–412
Computer-aided diagnosis
  in mammography, 316
  in ultrasonography, 310
Contrast agents, for lymph node sonography, 377
Core-needle biopsy, 327–333, 377–378
Coronal plane, in three-dimensional (volume)
  ultrasonography, 392, 394–395, 397
Cortical morphology, in lymph node sonography,
  371–372
Cysts, gel, in implant rupture, 363

D

Deflation, of implants, 357–358
Digital technology, 300
Doppler evaluation, 308
Drop-away sign, of implant rupture, 360–361

E

Elasticity, tissue, 308–310
Elastography, 301, 308–310, **407–415**
  clinical studies of, 412, 414–415
  principles of, 407–408
  shear wave, 408–409, 412
  static (compression), 408, 410–412

F

False ceiling sign, of implant rupture, 361
Field-of-view imaging, extended, 301–302
Filled-fold sign, of implant rupture, 361
Fine-needle aspiration biopsy, 327–333, 377
Four-dimensional imaging, 302
Frequency compounding, for speckle reduction, 303

G

Gel bleed, from implants, 359–360
Granuloma, silicone, in implant rupture, 361, 363

Ultrasound Clin 6 (2011) 417–419
doi:10.1016/S1556-858X(11)00085-5

H

Harmonic imaging, 306–308
Hilum, appearance of, for lymph node sonography, 371

I

Implants, **345–368**
    clinical history of, 349
    contraction and calcification of, 346
    evaluation of, 347–349
    fillers for, 345–346
    placement of, 345
    scanning for
        double-lumen, 356–357
        failure of, 357–361
        normal appearance in, 353–357
        pitfalls in, 361
        single-lumen saline-filled, 355–356
        single-lumen silicone gel-filled, 355–356
        technique for, 349–353
    silicone, 361–367
    types of, 345
Interactive volume cube, in three-dimensional ultrasonography, 387–388
Invasive lobular carcinoma, **313–325**
    axillary lymph node metastasis from, 320–321
    clinical features of, 315
    comparative imaging methods for, 322–323
    epidemiology of, 313–314
    magnetic resonance imaging for, 321–323
    mammographic features of, 315–318, 322–323
    metastasis from, 315, 320–321
    pathology of, 314
    subtypes of, 314
    ultrasound appearances of, 318–320

L

Lobular carcinoma, invasive. See Invasive lobular carcinoma.
Lymph node sonography, **369–380**
    contrast agents for, 377
    cortical morphology in, 371–372
    echogenicity in, 372–373
    for implants, 351–352
    for invasive lobular carcinoma, 320–321
    for lymphoma, 375–376
    for metastatic cancer, 375
    for percutaneous biopsy, 377–378
    for sentinel node biopsy, 376–377
    hilum and, 371
    normal anatomy in, 369–370
    pathophysiology of, 370–373
    patterns of, 373–375
    shape of nodes in, 371
    silicone in, 362–363
        size of nodes in, 370–371
        vascular patterns in, 373
Lymphoma, 375–376

M

Magnetic resonance imaging
    for breast implants, 347–348
    for invasive lobular carcinoma, 321–323
Mammography
    for calcifications, 335–336
    for invasive lobular carcinoma, 315–318, 322–323
Metastasis
    from invasive lobular carcinoma, 315, 320–321
    to lymph nodes, 375
Miniaturization, of systems, 300
Multiplanar display, in three-dimensional ultrasonography, 386–387
Multislide display, in three-dimensional ultrasonography, 387

N

Navigation, in three-dimensional ultrasonography, 388–389

P

Peak-and-trough appearance, as artifact, 365
Percutaneous biopsy, of lymph nodes, 377–378
Phase aberration correction, 301
Pleomorphic lobular carcinoma, 314
Probes, 300–301, 404–405
Pseudo-debris, in implant, 363
Pseudo-line sign, as artifact, 363, 365
Pseudo-standard double-lumen appearance, as artifact, 363, 365
Pseudo–wavy-line sign, in implant rupture, 364

R

Rupture, of implants, 346, 359–361, 364

S

Saline implants
    failure of, 357–361
    scanning for, normal appearance of, 353–357
Sentinel lymph node biopsy, 376–377
Shaded surface-rendered display, in three-dimensional ultrasonography, 387
Shear wave elastography, 408–409, 412
Shell pattern, in normal implant, 363
Signet ring lobular carcinoma, 314
Silicone
    in implants
        failure of, 357–361

normal appearance of, 353–357
  in soft tissue, 361–367
Sine sign, of implant rupture, 360–361
Snowstorm appearance, of implant, 363
Spatial compounding, 301, 303–305
Speckle processing, 301
Speckle reduction, 302–306
Speed of sound, correction for, 302
Spiculation
  differential diagnosis of, 395
  in invasive lobular carcinoma, 317
Static (compression) elastography, 408, 410–412
Stepladder sign, of implant rupture, 360–361

T

Temporal compounding, for speckle reduction,
  302–303
Terminal ductal lobular unit, in three-dimensional
  ultrasonography, 390–392
Three-dimensional (volume) ultrasonography, 302,
  381–406
  advantages of, 399–402
  anatomic correlation in, 389–393
  applications of, 398
  automated data acquisition in, 383
  calibrated probe for, 404–405
  coronal plane in, 392, 394–395, 397

data acquisition in, 382–384
definition of, 381–383
disadvantages of, 402–403
evolution of, 382
for benign lesions, 398–399
for malignant lesions, 399
image analysis in, 386, 398
image display in, 385–389
image optimization in, 384
image processing in, 384–385
image review in, 395–396
pitfalls in, 403
protocol for, 403–404
workflow issues in, 403
Tissue elasticity, 308–310
Tissue harmonic imaging, 306–308
Transmit gain control, 300

V

Vascular patterns, in lymph node sonography, 373
Virtual rescan, in three-dimensional ultrasonography,
  388–389
Volume ultrasonography. See Three-dimensional
  (volume) ultrasonography.

W

Wavy-line sign, in implant rupture, 360–361, 364

Printed and bound by CPI Group (UK) Ltd, Croydon, CR0 4YY

03/10/2024

01040351-0014